For the Love of Occupation

REFLECTIONS ON A CAREER IN OCCUPATIONAL THERAPY

MILDRED ROSS, OTR/L, FAOTA

AOTA PRESS

The American
Occupational Therapy
Association, Inc.

Vision Statement
The American Occupational Therapy Association advances occupational therapy as the pre-eminent profession in promoting the health, productivity, and quality of life of individuals and society through the therapeutic application of occupation.

Mission Statement
The American Occupational Therapy Association advances the quality, availability, use, and support of occupational therapy through standard-setting, advocacy, education, and research on behalf of its members and the public.

AOTA Centennial Vision
We envision that occupational therapy is a powerful, widely recognized, science-driven, and evidence-based profession with a globally connected and diverse workforce meeting society's occupational needs.

AOTA Staff
Frederick P. Somers, *Executive Director*
Christopher M. Bluhm, *Chief Operating Officer*

Chris Davis, *Director, AOTA Press*
Ashley Hofmann, *Production Editor*
Victoria Davis, *Editorial Assistant*

Beth Ledford, *Director, Marketing and Member Communications*
Emily Harlow, *Technology Marketing Specialist*
Jennifer Folden, *Marketing Specialist*

The American Occupational Therapy Association, Inc.
4720 Montgomery Lane
Bethesda, MD 20814
Phone: 301-652-AOTA (2682)
TDD: 800-377-8555
Fax: 301-652-7711
www.aota.org
To order: 1-877-404-AOTA (2682)

Disclaimers
This publication is designed to provide accurate and authoritative information in regard to the subject matter covered. It is sold or distributed with the understanding that the publisher is not engaged in rendering legal, accounting, or other professional service. If legal advice or other expert assistance is required, the services of a competent professional person should be sought.
—From the Declaration of Principles jointly adopted by the American Bar Association and a
    Committee of Publishers and Associations

It is the objective of the American Occupational Therapy Association to be a forum for free expression and interchange of ideas. The opinions expressed by the contributor to this work are her own and not necessarily those of the American Occupational Therapy Association.

ISBN 10: 1-56900-244-4
ISBN 13: 978-1-56900-244-5

Library of Congress: #2009922285

Design by Sarah E. Ely, Michael Melletz
Composition by Shepherd, Inc., Dubuque, IA; Michael Melletz, Germantown, MD
Printed by Automated Graphics Systems, Inc., White Plains, MD

In loving memory of my dear parents,
Sarah Leah and Harry Lovit

With love and admiration for my adult children,
Susan, Eric, and Sara-Ann; her husband Bobby;
and son Nathan

To my sister Hadis, her husband Herman Baren,
their son Lionel Baren, his wife Edwina, their daughter Esther,
and her husband Tom Kellam

In memoriam, Dr. Frederick Marcus Brown III
March 31, 1948–September 7, 2008

CONTENTS

ACKNOWLEDGMENTS

My immense gratitude is extended to Marilyn Cole Schiraldi, OTR/L, MS, FAOTA, for her persistence in encouraging me to write this story. She provided guidance and edited two earlier drafts. Marli understood that it was important to me to express how, in my ordinary daily life, my clients, friends, family, and mentors provided extraordinary influence that greatly enriched me. There were so many issues to discuss, and having her wise mind to guide me helped clarify the direction I needed to take.

It was necessary to have people other than occupational therapists read my material to be sure it could be readily understood, despite the specific subject matter. I am very grateful for the substantial counsel my editor and friend Roberta J. Buland gave me on an early outline and draft. My brother-in-law Herman Baren, folk poet Shirley Hodes, Rosalind Richman, and Cathy Smith also are not associated with occupational therapy. They reviewed the manuscript with keen objectivity and provided helpful suggestions.

All the people I mention in the text have left a monumental mark on me. I am grateful for their friendship, generosity of spirit, and acceptance. Three friends in particular have mentored me for the longest time of all: Valnere McLean, OTR/L, MS, FAOTA; Brenda Smaga, OTR/L, MS, FAOTA; and Marcus Brown, PhD.

Early in my career, Valnere and Brenda encouraged my writing and edited my manuscripts carefully. They continue to be a wonderful source. In doing so, they raised me to a higher level of thought and improvement. I appreciate them with a full heart. My friendship with Marcus, a clinical psychologist, began in a state psychiatric hospital 30 years ago. He was for me a resource of knowledge in geriatrics and in my development of the Five-Stage Group Model.

I have learned from and feel beholden to the occupational therapists I have known in the Connecticut Occupational Therapy Association, and I feel for each of them a very great affection and gratitude. I am indebted to and appreciative of the assistance of AOTA Press director Chris Davis and production editors, Tim Sniffin, Ashley Hofmann, and Victoria Davis in getting this book published.

In 1999, as a precursor to writing about clients, I wrote an article in *Advance for Occupational Therapy* called, "My Client, My Mentor," which is presented with permission in revised form in Chapter 4. That article attests to my lasting appreciation for my connection with clients, from whom there can be much to learn about strength of spirit. My sense of compassion deepened over time because of them. I learned too that, although I could not control outcome, when I brought respect, warmth, and a sense of enjoyment to the treatment process, I felt a connection between us.

INTRODUCTION

Occupational therapy addresses the physical, cognitive, psychosocial, sensory, and other aspects of performance in a variety of contexts to support engagement in everyday life activities that affect health, well-being, and quality of life (American Occupational Therapy Association [AOTA], 2004). Occupational therapy services can promote health and wellness "to people who have or are at risk for developing an illness, injury, disease, disorder, condition, impairment, disability, activity limitation, or participation restriction" (AOTA, 2008, p. 673).

The *occupation* in occupational therapy does not refer to vocational training; rather, it encompasses all of the essential daily tasks or the components of a routine that people perform to create a meaningful lifestyle (AOTA, 2008). The focus of occupational therapy intervention is in accomplishing *activities of daily living (ADLs),* which start with getting up in the morning and preparing oneself for the day, and meeting the demands of *instrumental activities of daily living (IADLs),* which are complex tasks that support the individual's life roles—successfully engaging in education, embracing one's chosen work, enabling age-appropriate play, achieving engagement in chosen leisure pursuits, and promoting the full spectrum of social interaction that is important at any age.

Occupational therapy professionals work with people who have difficulty performing for themselves what is required in vital areas. Occupational therapists use the individual's choice of purposeful tasks to provide treatment that is based on learning by doing, changing by practicing, and becoming by achieving. Therapists find solutions that keep people independent and living a life that feels balanced and satisfying.

The study of occupational therapy teaches practitioners to evaluate an individual's needs. The therapist selects, analyzes, and sequences a task as it relates to the focus of intervention. Therapists learn to train people in useful motor skills that have been hampered by a faulty health process or injury. For example, to perform their best, school children might need help with listening skills, legible writing, or personal organization. Patients in a hospital or recovering at home might need to learn to dress themselves, prepare food, or accomplish other homemaking tasks they now must do differently. Adults admitted into day care settings can benefit from special exercises and specific sensory stimulation. The therapist uses a background in anatomy, physiology, neurology, and behavioral science in preparation for teaching those skills.

One need not be sick to feel better and do better! Occupational therapy also offers preventative intervention that can accommodate and adapt the individual's strengths for a continuation of health when circumstances threaten that health (Baker, 2007; Clark et al., 1997; Jackson, Carlson, Mandel, Zemke, & Clark, 1998). This can translate into working with the changing needs of healthy elderly people in the community or an assisted-living setting. Therapists can work with parents who need help at home with learning how to hold, feed, or play with their children who are at risk. Therapists also are valuable and necessary in industrial settings, where they can offer instruction on ergonomics and the readjustment of task performance.

When dysfunction occurs at birth or in the early years, therapeutic intervention helps guide development by supporting position and movement and by offering appropriate stimulation. Adaptations might be required for older people who need to learn to use assistive devices or require alterations in the environment that make it easier to perform necessary tasks.

For healing after orthopedic surgery, the skills of an occupational therapy professional usually are required. Physicians' and therapists' protocols can include guidelines for special types of splints to be created, mobilization of joints and soft tissue, thermal modalities, precautions, and retraining for functional use. Occupational therapists might choose hand therapy, for example, as a specialty.

Sometimes treatment requires a readiness program. People might first require increased strengthening, sensory stimulation, and endurance to become motivated to consider meaningful occupations in their lives. Occupational therapy is sensitive to these needs as it evaluates the need to make the transition from dependence to independence in important, useful tasks. That transformation might occur in a group home for people with chronic disabilities, in a school, or in work services and rehabilitation programs outside hospitals. Staff consultation, hands-on demonstration, and direct treatment of the person might be necessary.

As I reflected on the way to which I had attended my practice in occupational therapy—incorporating my increased appreciation, insights, and growth, as well as the changes within the profession—I came to believe the following philosophy: To promote client participation, the occupational therapist takes the time to understand how to create the goals of therapy with the client. That process encompasses the client's hopes and available strengths, the culture, and particular environmental constraints. Trust and empathy are important in the relationship, putting an altruistic spin on intervention, but they also distinguish occupational therapy from other health care professions. The occupational therapy professional seeks compatibility of the intervention goals with the client's physical, emotional, cognitive, and spiritual needs and attributes to ensure a client-centered approach. The therapist is uniquely placed for that task because of training in physical disabilities, psychiatry, the biological sciences, and psychology (AOTA, 2008).

In her address at the Columbia University occupational therapy commencement in 2005, Janet Krauthamer (2005) said, "Our role, as occupational therapists, is to help enable our clients to feel this sense of accomplishment, to feel that they, in fact, have done it themselves" (p. 6). That is the empowerment that is possible and distinctive to occupational therapy practitioners.

Occupational therapy often fills the gap in a person's healing when it falls between the end of acute illness and the beginning of adjustment to a new, productive life. No other profession fills that space as completely. That link—that quality of service—cannot be overlooked in the healing process. It is that essential.

This book describes the familiar, traditional places where occupational therapy professionals have functioned, particularly where this author has been, but occupational therapists have gone beyond the places recounted here to all corners of the globe, most remarkably into developing nations (see Appendix; also Kronenberg, Algado, & Pollard, 2005). Moreover, occupational therapists are found in a variety of institutions, in prisons, in industry, and in different kinds of shelters. Many are using technology in extraordinary, creative ways. They work anywhere social distress, medical issues, or uncommon conditions exist so that people who need to live with greater independence can obtain the skills and habits to make that possible.

All along in my practice in occupational therapy during the half-century beginning in 1951, I witnessed a range of emotions in the challenged lives of clients as we worked together—from denial to determined acceptance of their predicaments. Motivation to help themselves came from different sources. Although techniques and treatments change as knowledge increases—and the pace does appear more hectic now—people's needs, fears, joys, and expectations are timeless and universal.

My use of narratives to describe occupational therapy clients is intended to show that much can be learned from them and that those lessons can be shared with others. When unexpected suffering occurs in people's lives, they must move mountains, turning submission into sublime acceptance, or choose to struggle endlessly with change. These narratives are placed within the context of a 50-year career, and they reflect the influence of the times as seen through my eyes.

The story of traditional occupational therapy practice during that period is instructive, and the stories of clients and the mentors I have met along the way illustrate the conflicts and joys that exist in occupational therapy practice but cannot be learned from textbooks. Sometimes family members undermine treatment, or other therapists intrude to cause conflict. Especially important are the unexpected ups and downs that must be endured and survived during a career. A therapist meets unplanned occurrences that hamper or improve individual or group sessions, learns to redirect anger or inappropriate behavior, and often assumes the role of advocate—all the while managing personal emotional involvement that arises in the work. Those were the challenges that kept me engrossed and encouraged me to continue in practice.

Like many in the health care professions, occupational therapists are affected by public policy, medical breakthroughs, bureaucratic pitfalls, cultural and historical occurrences, and inspired colleagues. Most of the chapters that follow begin with my reflections on the major social and political events of each decade. The mood, style, spirit, and needs of each era are distinctive, and occupational therapy practice responded to them with change and growth. Reviewing the past can be a forward-looking exercise because it can help to shape the future. In 1951, my work in occupational therapy began, when the return of so many injured World War II veterans sparked a demand for research that would result in better drugs and new treatment methods overall (Padilla, 2005a). For the first time it was possible to treat a population of patients that had been unreachable. And with the new possibility of working with those patients, the need for occupational therapists was growing. I had a wide range of positions from which to choose.

My involvement in the profession also offered me the freedom to find a personal interest that few pursued and no one wrote about very much. This was a good lesson to learn; it gave me an opportunity to find my own passion or *bliss,* as some call it. The path would take me into the world of group therapy with a population not usually exposed to it. Pursuing this personal interest helped me flourish and create a professional niche.

It also reflected the growing interest in society for group member interaction. When I attended Columbia University, the study of group dynamics was not in the occupational therapy curriculum. But in the decades that followed, workshops and eventually courses became part of that curriculum. Interest in teaching and learning about the central nervous system also grew, and I came to appreciate the interconnection of all the systems in the body that influence and contribute to human behavior. All this went into the development of my own approach to facilitating group work. The spirit of the times greatly influenced my actions.

I received abundant help at key times from very good people who often became friends. I learned from their competence, generosity, and kindness, and I appreciate them even today.

An interesting tenet of occupational therapy is the usefulness of storytelling, particularly as a review of one's early life (Clark, 1993; Hasselkus, 2002). Early influences of key people, recollection of the choices I made, and sharp experiences in my formative years seeded my choices and aptitude for my later work. I discuss my personal life only briefly because I want to keep the focus on the narratives of others and on the changes that occur in work and practice, which is the purpose of this book.

How anyone ends up in later years, emotionally and spiritually, from a career is as important a consideration as what our financial investments will pay in retirement. I can describe from my perspective how much the occupational therapy profession nourishes innovation and service to others even as it replenishes the therapist. I extended myself to others, learning what was meaningful and helpful, and that has influenced my personal growth. Experiencing the people I met nurtures the rest of my life.

My wish is that those who read these stories come away with appreciation for the remarkable meaningfulness of the "occupation" in occupational therapy and, thereby, in the lives of people. As occupational therapy approaches its 100th year as a profession (AOTA, 2007), it is my hope that, by looking back at just one occupational therapist's career path, readers will find something of themselves and their own clients in my story and perhaps chronicle their own journey in diverse ways that remind us all of the importance of occupation.

chapter 1

MY FAMILY:
"THE LONG WAY IS THE SHORT WAY"

It often is true that the apple does not fall far from the tree. My parents greatly influenced my actions and beliefs. I observed them very carefully as a child, and I thought about their messages to me.

I saw that my mother handled all financial affairs and appeared to be the decision maker; my father seemed indecisive and spent as much time as he could at his writing and reading. He expressed to me a few times the wish that his many translations of English classics into Hebrew and his original writings might be published, but that was never realized. He never pursued it in an active way. His short, stocky frame bent over his notebooks by the hour was a familiar sight to me. A wide gap in communication seemed to exist between the adult and my child's worlds. Posture and body language sometimes were the only important elements I could learn from when thinking about him and other adults.

My father was a lifelong, self-taught student who spent much of his waking hours reading philosophy, poetry, and history when he was not teaching the Hebrew language to Jewish school children. He would render brief, lofty statements to me. When I complained about a friend, he would say, "If someone asks you for something, give it to him." This helped me feel guilty when I was not generous. Or, when he saw me studying, and I complained about a grade, he would say, "You should not read a history book like a novel." This had better results; I began to think about his meaning and to create my own self-help devices. My grades improved. However, not all of his enigmatic messages were that easy to solve. He would say, "I fear tomorrow will be a nice day." I took a while to decipher that, to him, *fear* meant *awe*—as in the fear of God—and in that context, fear meant that he *appreciated the possibility* of a nice day. He frequently said, like an affirmation, "The long way is the short way," always insisting on giving time to ensure the quality of one's labor.

Three times a day, at specific hours, my father prayed. He loved and consistently observed all the rituals of religion, stating their purpose was to remind him of his constant gratitude to God for his life. However, he strongly believed, and reinforced often to me, that it was ethics and morality, the beliefs and the behavior, in religious teachings that counted the most. We must be consistently honest and contribute to the welfare of others. Also, although I saw his acceptance of diverse beliefs and different kinds of people in all his actions, I did not doubt his loyalty to Judaism. He was easily ruffled by daily vicissitudes; in fact, he often was reduced to helplessness about what action he should take. Faithful prayer must have helped him maintain some inner stability in the face of events he could not control.

My father retained his belief that one sentence says it all even when his judgment, memory, and ambulatory powers failed. When he was about 100 years old and living in a nursing home, I frequently went to attend to him. He often did not recognize me, and I sought means to stimulate him and jog his memory. One day as I pushed his wheelchair into the courtyard of the facility, I pointed out to him two pigeons strutting in front of us. I was anxious to focus his attention and called out, "Look papa, two pigeons are walking ahead of us, a brother and a sister!" A sparkle spread over his lackluster eyes as he leaned forward to examine the pair while suggesting, "And why not two lovers?"

My father, in accordance with doctrine, honored a strict obligation to teach the Hebrew Bible daily to my sister and me individually. My sister, Hadis, is 3 years older than me. She absorbed all of my father's training and served as his helper by reviewing lessons with his students from the time she was 9 years old. Hadis also has a magnificent, melodious voice that never failed to thrill me throughout my childhood. I loved attending the programs my father arranged for the general congregation to demonstrate the progress the Hebrew school was making, and she was his star, carrying the entire production. She greatly brightened our circumstances, our crowded apartment with its makeshift furniture and emphasis on frugality, with her glorious voice. She exposed me to her innate love of classical music. Despite skimpy funds when we were in grade school, my parents always found the money for piano and singing lessons for Hadis, because her musical talent was so evident, and for tap-dancing and piano lessons for me, so that I should not feel less worthy.

From the age of 4 until I was 14, I studied with my father. I did not enjoy the sessions because he was impatient with my questions and slow understanding. Unlike my sister, I continued to resist my father's instruction—much to my regret now—but I always enjoyed the times he stopped a lesson to tell me his point of view or to offer an interesting assessment of some matter. This never was often enough for me because I needed the personal interaction.

Despite my father's intense drive for self-study and the general respect he obtained from others for the knowledge he would demonstrate, he was insecure and frustrated. He indulged in impulsive rages that were terrifying to me. If I became the object of his rage, I was safe only if my mother were present. She would interrupt the outburst, although then his anger often was redirected at her but only with words. I learned something from that and, when I was older, I began to use defiance with him, finally stating emphatically that I would never allow him to raise his hand to me again. My feelings of ambivalence toward him grew as I realized how different he was when he would share his thoughts with me or take me on a trip with him. Then, he could be warm and kind.

Thinking about matters by myself, I believe, helped me develop a necessary tolerance for living with the uncertainty and confusion that was abundant everywhere. It was the era of the Great Depression. Pottsville, Pennsylvania, where I was raised, was a small town with a growing suburb. We lived in town with the most recent wave of immigrants and people who had no money to move to the suburbs. We also needed to live close to the synagogue so that my father could walk there and not have to drive on the Sabbath as our scripture directed.

There was no talk of religion, politics, or—heaven forefend—sex. When I forced a question, I generally was told I "did not need to know anything about any of it." We were expected to behave in rigidly prescribed ways. Elders and teachers in the community would remind us. Timidly, I usually stayed in line, often not understanding but burying my resentments. I did notice that rich people or educated people with titles were respected regardless of their behavior. I saw an advantage to education and to gaining that status.

The homes of my friends were not too much different from my own. My friends and I had a great time pooling our bits of knowledge, observations, and misinformation with the natural result of creating more misinformation, heightened fears, uneasy emotions, and more confusion. Thank heavens for the availability of my friends' older siblings. They revealed the possibility of a freer life. As young adults, they assisted our progress toward maturity when they gave us extra money for movies and magazines. Their rakish behavior fascinated me because they escaped punishment, for example, for engaging in sexual activity or breaking the Sabbath rules.

My mother was firm on tradition and propriety, but she also was very patient, quite pragmatic, and a good listener. She always took my side, sometimes compromising her own belief. Her kind of love was unconditional loyalty. She was clear on her principles. Among the most important was her insistence on scrupulous cleanliness. She lived to be 105, and to the end of her days, she radiated freshness. However, learning from her befuddled me. She would answer my questions with, "I can't tell you exactly how to do that; you have to watch me and see what I do." When I wanted to cook, she might say, "To make this, take a handful of flour, an egg, an egg full of water, and a pinch of spice and mix it to the consistency you like." She would substitute one ingredient for another in a recipe. Sometimes the substitution worked, and sometimes it did not. I favor her in this way. Her life was so full of constraining realities that it was only in the kitchen that she could exercise the luxury of options and risk taking.

My mother always put the needs of others ahead of her own and worked from morning to night, cooking, cleaning, and responding to anyone's need for her help. She supplemented my father's earnings by feeding and cleaning up after strangers who found respite in our home on a daily basis. The Jewish community paid her for this service as they supported unemployed Jews, as well as those of other faiths, who traveled from town to town during the Depression, looking for work. Some of them were hobos, but there also were upstanding, religious people earning their living by collecting for Jewish charities. A maxim of the Jewish religion is that we are all responsible for each other's welfare, so we must help the stranger.

Life was very demanding of my mother, but I never heard her complain. It was a message of total selflessness that could not clarify for me what I deserved from life. There was never time to share feelings or to feel that feelings even mattered! Yet in some odd way, she conveyed to my sister and me that we, her children, should expect more than she had without revealing how this could come about for us. We all have seen the television advertisements with the beautiful model saying confidently, "I must have this because I deserve it." Mother accepted the status quo for herself. She would have said, "Not for myself, but my children deserve more."

My sister and I never doubted that we were loved greatly. My mother would hug and kiss us often. For years, she appeared in the bedroom of our cold-water flat early in the morning carrying the small oil stove so we would awake to warmth. A hot breakfast always was ready for us. Her thoughtfulness was endless. When I got a rash on my legs from my woolen snow pants, she sewed soft linings in them, and when I cried she was sympathetic.

My father was less demonstrative but showed his caring in another way. I have a vivid memory of his indisputably perfect potato latkes. He would kiss me on the forehead and invite me to taste them immediately. He loved ice cream but would never have it unless a good portion could be afforded for all. Those times made me feel very happy. In retrospect, it seems that much of the message of love was couched in the presentation of food.

Life was not always confined to our village. My mother was the second of eight siblings, most of whom lived in New York City. We would visit my grandmother there, staying for a very lengthy visit at least once a year. On those occasions, each of my aunts and uncles or their spouses would take my sister and me to museums, planetariums, theaters, or concerts. When we were children, we would go to the beautiful parks in New York, to the surrounding beaches, or to visit relatives. My Uncle Moe, who traveled the globe as a civil engineer in government service, would bring us native jewelry, handmade from beads and plants. Relatives sent us beautiful books to read, crafts to make, and big dolls that we loved. My aunts and uncles are indelibly impressed in my memory as loving, kind, and very creative people who enriched the lives of my immediate small family.

Both parents expressed themselves in cryptic ways, and their speech often became a code for me to decipher. Indeed, when I later learned more about the influence of culture, historical experience, and personality on the style of communication, I understood that this was a learned practice of theirs. One protected oneself by remaining cryptic. Many of the different nationalities I met in clinical practice are like this, too.

My parents were products of a ghetto in Russia where there was very little trust in what was outside it. A question was responded to with another question or an ambiguous answer. They had learned that the simplest response might be misunderstood and then trouble could ensue. It was necessary to gauge what was safe to reveal, even to friends.

I listened and watched my parents closely for a key word or accompanying action to reveal the intent of their remarks. Because there was so little open discussion, I watched them closely to see whether they were sad, worried, happy, or planning something. So few questions were answered clearly. The notion that I had to look beyond words for clarification might have influenced the way I would learn about people in the future. It could be the reason I am attracted to working with people who do not reveal themselves through speech. Their silence reinforced my ability to study body language and other nonverbal cues for a greater understanding of what was really going to happen when adults spoke.

Until the end of their days, both of my parents remained unworldly and found it difficult to carry on negotiations with others. As a child, I realized they somehow were out of step with others in our small community. However, I also saw that they were respected. They consistently demonstrated a repertoire of positive, compelling actions of total honesty and generosity in their contacts with others. They always displayed courage in their actions and persisted honorably when performing work and meeting obligations. Both worked into their 80s, my father conducting religious services on the Sabbath or at holiday times for small groups of isolated Jewish families and my mother supporting his efforts by traveling with him when necessary. Their overall conduct remained rooted in their staunch belief in prayer, cleanliness, and good works. That behavioral trilogy had a fundamental influence on me. They accepted their lifelong struggle and their poverty, never showing envy or bitterness. And this made them an anomaly. They were totally without guile. Their deep sense of responsibility and meekness lingers in me. Whatever the task, whether it was scrubbing or it was praying, both parents attended to it fully, treating it as important work. That was the power that kept them from feeling completely discouraged whenever dire circumstances occurred in their lives.

When I graduated from high school, my family moved from Pennsylvania to Hartford, Connecticut. We lived in a neglected neighborhood where my father found some meager religious work to do. I understood that unless I had more education, I would remain there forever. At first, my father would not agree with my determination to attend college, but when I insisted, and my mother encouraged me, he accepted my decision. His income from teaching and his work as a sexton was little, so without discussion, he supplemented it by quietly getting another job as a dishwasher and stock clerk because he had no other marketable skills. At that time, he was in his early 60s. The only local four-year college was St. Joseph College, a Catholic college, but he reflected that my attendance there would be broadening for me.

As usual, my father did not discuss his personal feelings about his new work, but I got the impression that he did not please his supervisors because he worked very slowly, as thoroughly and carefully as he would work when he performed his religious duties. Those were not desirable traits in a dishwasher or stock clerk. As he related humorously to us the events of his day, I thought many of them were heartbreaking, because his supervisors gave him very little respect. One event especially tickled my father. It seemed that every chance he had, such as at break times, he would rush to find a place where he might sit and open a book to read. A kindred spirit noticed this and approached him with curiosity. "What are you doing, Harry?" asked the man.

"I'm praying," answered my father.

"Well, for whom are you praying?" continued the man.

"I'm praying for you, I'm praying for me, I'm praying for the whole world," responded my father.

Deadpanned his new friend, "Well, Harry, can we rely on you?" His coworker, by questioning with humor and irony my father's hopes, beliefs, and blind faith in the face of daily hardships that both of them knew, amused my father greatly.

Because money for school was scarce, I studied hard to accumulate sufficient credits to complete college in three years. When I graduated with a bachelor of science in 1946 and began looking for work, the possibilities discouraged me. I experimented with being a secretary and a salesperson, and found no pleasure in them. About two years later, I went to New York City where I eventually enrolled at Columbia University to study occupational therapy. My sister Hadis, who after World War II was employed by the famous Fuller Brush Company, earned what was then considered excellent pay: $65 a week. She was faithful in sending a weekly stipend to me, generously and kind-heartedly supporting my efforts.

Before I entered Columbia, I had placed a newspaper ad for my services as a live-in babysitter. I had secured a room with kitchen privileges for my services. One time when I returned home to Connecticut for a visit, I lamented at length to my father that I was becoming too discouraged with school. Continuing was too hard for me. He listened for as long as I spoke and then uttered a single sentence, "What you need, Malka (my Hebrew name), is a shot of courage!" I laughed at his use of a medical metaphor. The look on his face made me feel understood. I knew he considered my schooling a commitment I had made. Because it was not pleasant or easy were not reasons to discontinue such a commitment. I returned to school.

My parents were not role models for risk taking. They had had all the adventure they ever needed immigrating to America and making their own way. They had a baggage of fears that also penetrated my consciousness. But their constant encouragement and pride in me smoothed over the fears they haplessly imparted. I always could be sure of their approval and regard for my welfare.

What my parents always gave me was enormous support. They gave their time, their possessions, and whatever assistance was requested. They never disparaged any adventure I wanted to undertake, not necessarily because they thought I would succeed, but because they felt their duty was to encourage my trying. It is popular today to believe that your child should have high ambitions. Their expectations always had been exceedingly modest, and they did not voice any great expectations for me. Their message to me was the unique value of their totally committed support. This message of support reinforced that the striving part was most important and to be sustained. Failure or rejections were not dishonorable.

I cherish a picture of my mother (circa 1910) sitting with a large group of her peers all outfitted in stiffly starched nurses' caps and gowns marking the completion of their first-year nursing studies. Unfortunately my mother could not return. Her mother, my grandmother, had become ill, requiring her to take care of her seven siblings as she was the oldest daughter. The theme (or maybe melody) of health care drifted down to me it seems.

Surely, my parents shaped me, but it is speculative to draw a straight line between my early life's influences and the path I eventually took. Nonetheless, it was inevitable that I would choose to serve others, to be attracted to and compassionate with people who were as confused and clueless as I had been, and to be content with the unpretentious settings where I worked for 50 years. I developed my own special interest in the profession I chose. I persisted during the last 25 years to explore and examine that interest with great thoroughness in writing articles and books about the Five-Stage Group Model (Ross, 1991, 1997). The method engages people—even if they are seriously regressed or nonverbal—in visibly enjoying being together in a meaningful way. I also realized my father's earlier ambitions to publish. I believe he would have liked that. Writing and sharing are laborious work for me, but my father's prescription, "the long way is the short way," provided insight about how to promote an essential program for those who otherwise might be ignored or forgotten.

chapter 2

THE 1950S:
STARTING OUT

OCCUPATIONAL THERAPY TRAINING

Completing My Internship

Columbia University had accepted my bachelor's degree, so in 1949 I entered the two-year certificate program in occupational therapy. Part of the training involved spending a nine-month internship working with patients in various settings with physical disabilities and psychiatric illnesses, as well as in a specialty setting such as a tuberculosis facility or a pediatric hospital. I chose the tuberculosis placement as part of my physical disability placement, and I worked at Haverstraw, a hospital that treated children with polio. My final internship was in 1950 at the Bronx Veteran's Hospital, a place that hummed with the influx of veterans from World War II.

At that time, all occupational therapy treatment was based on the medical model, and patients usually were treated only by referral from a physician (West, 1992). Veterans with a variety of disabilities were referred to our department. Those with prostheses to replace lost limbs needed to learn how to perform tasks in self-care, such as bathing and dressing, and to explore general vocational skills, which might include typing, carpentry, or other interests or skills. But there also were patients with paralysis or other neurological impairments that resulted from brain injuries. Brain trauma impairs the ability to learn and remember, and that internship introduced me to the real task of the occupational therapist: to be creative and adaptive in helping guide the individual to success. All tasks that make up the activities of daily living, or ADLs, had to be adapted to the abilities of the individual patient. We students and the veterans became comrades-in-arms as we learned from and taught one another how to face the smallest challenges of daily life. We were given a lot of time to converse, and we were allowed to provide hours at a time of individualized instruction to our clients whenever it was necessary.

Veterans with mental illness also were treated at the Bronx hospital. Students learned how to suggest and instruct in crafts—the list included weaving, carpentry, jig inventing, art and metal work, hand setting of type, glove making, and pottery—that could help control or relieve the symptoms of schizophrenia, mania, or depression. There was so much work to do that the hospital authorities encouraged students to continue working in the hospital beyond their internships, offering to pay for each month a student would stay.

It was a tremendous learning arena because the staff members were well trained and dedicated. I accepted the offer to stay on as a student and, much as I needed it, the pay seemed incidental to being happily challenged by the work.

Learning to Use a Cane

A momentous opportunity for me occurred during that field placement. It was there I met Peter Alverti, a hospital rehabilitation worker who treated the veterans who had lost their sight. He was himself totally blind, and he had such great sensitivity that he could negotiate all of New York City without using a special cane. I engaged him in conversations and began to regard him as a *mentor*—long before that term became fashionable. I understood the many disappointments he sustained as a result of the ignorance of the sighted world around him. I was impressed with Mr. Alverti and his work.

I received permission from my occupational therapy supervisor to be trained by Mr. Alverti in the use of cane travel. He was a cultured man, gifted on many levels, who always had bloody scratch marks on both hands from the amount of Braille reading he did. He taught me cane travel by challenging me to learn it blindfolded and to trust him. Once, when practicing, I did not anticipate a staircase, but he was prepared for me to miss it, and he was there to catch me. I was jostled but not hurt. When he recognized that I was shaken by this, he asked me, "Is life *so* sweet, Miss Lovit?" I did not answer, but somehow I felt as though he was asking himself that question, too, because of the many discouraging situations he had endured.

Mr. Alverti also taught me Braille and other skills that would be useful for work with blind people. He was patient and compassionate. I felt his respect and this gave me confidence. I was determined to work with people with visual problems when I returned to Connecticut.

Passing the required national registration examinations in occupational therapy in 1951, I acquired the initials *OTR* after my name, and I returned to Connecticut.

THE BLIND THAT LEAD THE SIGHTED

Finding Kindred Excitement and Skilled Supervision

When I returned to Connecticut, I intended to work with people who were blind. I introduced myself as a new occupational therapist to Stetson K. Ryan, the director of the Connecticut State Board of Education of the Blind. I began by describing the skills I had learned for use with the population he served. We talked with a kindred excitement about how occupational therapy might be applied.

Mr. Ryan, a tall, lanky Abraham Lincoln look-alike, regarded me intently. At the end of our interview, he smiled and told me that he and his staff already had discussed the possibility of acquiring the services of a staff occupational therapist even though they had never had one. It was providence! At our next meeting, I accepted a starting salary of $2,800 a year even though I knew other places were offering $3,200. My title was supervisor of home teachers. Perceptive, supportive, and a monumental teacher, Mr. Ryan became another strong mentor for me. I saw that he was available for all the staff and imparted exceedingly high standards in performance and ethics, which he modeled himself.

Mr. Ryan directed an array of services for all the entitled people throughout the state who were blind or whose vision was so low they were considered legally blind. The State Board of Education of the Blind occupied a huge office area, a library–committee meeting room, and a flourishing sales department area in the Connecticut State Office Building in Hartford.

I was given a desk and some space in the large office area where I joined the other professionals. There was a supervisor who provided services for blind adolescents—one for small children with visual impairments and another for special cases that did not fit easily into the other categories. Also occupying desks in this office were rehabilitation counselors who helped blind adults find employment in their communities.

To this day, there are small stores and kiosks in many state buildings where people who are legally blind sell drinks, candy, newspapers, and other items. Those jobs enable them to earn a living. The supervisor of this program rarely was at her desk because she traveled constantly to visit and troubleshoot for the different businesses in many office buildings throughout Connecticut.

In contrast to today's demand for concise case reports, occupational therapists in those days were expected to write detailed reviews of every contact with every client. Mr. Ryan would comment at length on my work during our regular supervision hours. He took my training very seriously. He did that not by questioning my decisions as an occupational therapist but by helping me expand my skills in interactions with clients and the community.

The home teachers I supervised were all blind women almost twice my age. Their enormous skills and my awareness of the burden blindness placed on them intimidated me. Mr. Ryan recognized my dilemma. Once, using a less-saintly technique, he discussed the teachers with me, allowing me to see very human pictures of their personae that would help me understand their needs and how I might be of assistance to them. Mr. Ryan understood me well and trusted me to understand his remarks—I needed to know the teachers were not saints on pedestals but regular folk with human qualities and very human needs. I did come away from our unusual meeting feeling more relaxed about how I would handle relationships with the teachers. I could expect the teachers to be fair with me, as I would be with them.

I realized that Mr. Ryan wanted me to succeed. He helped me feel safe when making mistakes. Quietly, he would ask, "Is all that effort you are making really necessary?" Then he would give me his version of what he would do, making it clear to me that complicated methods and a strenuous outpouring of effort could not accomplish more than a simpler, more realistic approach. He started me on the path of reflecting on style and method for handling knotty situations, although it would take a lifetime to get into the habit of simplifying solutions and staying realistic. He was an early proponent of working "smarter not harder" to solve the multitude of problems that crossed his desk each day.

Mr. Ryan's first assignment to me was to teach the cane travel technique to Viola Jaenicke, a home teacher of long tenure. This instruction would allow her to walk independently from her home to the drugstore and the mailbox, an activity that had been lost to her when family members were no longer available. Home teachers were provided with sighted guides only during their working hours. Her success with cane travel strengthened my relationship with her, and we remained friends throughout her life as she enlightened me with insights she would share. At that time, I was among the first in Connecticut to teach a formal procedure in using the white cane, thanks to my training with Mr. Alverti. When the School for the Blind incorporated cane travel technique into its curriculum, the need for my instruction decreased.

One day I was meeting with Mr. Ryan when his phone rang. I overheard the information he was given. I realized that a huge private estate, the Harkness Estate on Long Island Sound in New London, Connecticut, was being donated to the state's department of parks. As soon as he hung up, I impulsively asked whether we could use the facilities there for groups of our clients. He immediately agreed and, finding the funding, arranged for us to do this. Thereafter, we took many groups of blind people on week-long holidays to the estate. Home teachers would join us along with their sighted guides to help us sometimes. My sister Hadis would donate her time and often come to help me.

In the early part of the 20th century, guests visited the Harkness family, often coming on their yachts from New York City and other places on the Sound to attend afternoon picnics. They docked near the immense lawn where canvas tents and long tables were set up. It was a setting for an impressionist painter. Waiters from the nearby town were hired to serve them. Now, our groups were experiencing this lovely site with its enormous mansion, many beautiful cottages, its own solarium, and a magnificent private beach. When I sometimes went to shop for box lunches for my groups, the storekeepers told me stories of the special opulence with which life was lived, perhaps just 30 years earlier when America had its first economic aristocracy. Now, in the early 1950s, ours was the first group from the general population in Connecticut to visit this place of elegance and beauty. For me it seemed an ideal setting for an occupational therapist to provide meaningful interventions. We worked on leisure skills like crafts or games and necessary activities like making beds and cooking, but mostly rest and relaxation were emphasized for those who had more difficult routines when they went back home.

At Harkness, we often took our guests to swim at the large private beach or to sit on the luxurious boardwalk while I read to them. One beautiful afternoon, I was reading a story by Guy de Maupassant that had a particularly descriptive passage about two people traveling on a train. One was a thirsty young man and the other a young wet nurse whose breasts were filling up with no prospect of imminent relief. The story describes the way the two characters met each other's needs. This was in the early 1950s, and I was in my mid-20s. I became embarrassed and unable to go on. I stopped and, taking advantage of my audience, I said, "Oh, my goodness, the wind just took that last page away." I had to make up a new version for the ending, but at least one of my friends was not fooled. A week later, I visited her in her home. Eleanor was an artist who had lost her sight in middle age because of diabetes. She said to me, "I know the story you were reading. So did the page really blow away?" She knew that in the story, the young man had assuaged his thirst by nursing at the breast of the wet nurse in a very natural way.

It may seem quaint now, but it did not at the time; such subjects were not discussed in polite conversation. There were formalities and courtesies that required we address everyone as Miss, Mrs., or Mr., because to use first names would imply an intrusive familiarity. I was used to it, so I was comfortable complying with behavior that nowadays might seem standoffish.

The Harkness estate and the beach have changed considerably during the past 50 years. Harkness would become regulated, formulated, and relegated to state department management. It is now the most sought-after camp for a variety of groups of people with disabilities. Building to support that purpose has altered its pristine beauty from when we first used it but made it more accommodating for many more people with different kinds of disabilities.

In my department at the board, the seven home teachers and their guides visited blind adults in their homes throughout Connecticut, educating them in how to manage almost every aspect of their lives. Those home teachers were prime examples of people who had adapted to living with blindness and were bringing their empathy and expertise to the newly blind. I would read each home teacher's typed report for each visit to determine whether clients required further attention. We were urged to intensify our outreach whenever and wherever possible to help us identify and provide whatever service would make life more comfortable for people with blindness. I also took referrals from other staff to visit clients in their homes when occupational therapy might be useful, and I did this covering the whole state.

I remember visiting an elderly client, happily making her aware of tax credits her blindness allowed her and about which she had not known but needed. I spent a week living with another elderly woman who was completely blind and whose move to a new apartment required acclimation to her new setting without assistance from her family. There was no family member available to help. Those clients demonstrated great fortitude to me. Today there is much less help available, and the new approach to services feels skimpy to me. I saw many courageous people who continually impressed me with their deep appreciation of services.

Clients taught by the home teachers from the Connecticut State Board of Education for the Blind could learn to sew, knit, or make craft items at home for sale throughout the state through the board's Sales Department and at special sites, such as the Trades Department. The latter was a residence and a sheltered workshop for blind people. The school for the blind, Oakhill; the Board of Education for the Blind; and the Trades Department were independent agencies that maintained a useful connection with one another. Many things have changed over the years, and the Sales Department no longer exists. Many blind children now have the opportunity to be mainstreamed through the public schools, and the school has altered its character as well. The philosophy of raising people born with poor or no sight has changed to promote more individual self-reliance and to offer new possibilities.

Forming a Lifelong Relationship With a Mentor

I formed lifelong relationships with many of the staff and the teachers. One colleague, Dorothea Simpson, was an English teacher turned social worker who became my permanent mentor. When she reached her 40s, Dorothea had decided to leave her teaching position and return to Smith College for a degree in social work. At the board, she worked with adolescents with visual impairments and their parents. We shared many personal hours despite the disparity in our ages. Once I lamented to her about feeling that I may not be doing enough, that I might be missing many ways to be useful to those I saw with difficulties. She responded that all one needed was ordinary intelligence and interest to succeed. The opportunity to examine with Dorothea what lay behind my fears led me to recognize my fundamental pain and regret I felt when working with blind people—especially those who could not accept their condition. The positive side is that alongside the strong emotions regarding blindness is the good feeling that both the client who is blind and the therapist can experience in the accomplishment of successful action taken. There was achievement and growth in acceptance on the part of many I will describe. I worked through many emotional times with Dorothea's help.

Teaching Mr. Snider to Weave While I Learned Marketing

Mr. Ryan stayed attuned to my strengths and helped me flourish. At another time during my first year, he assigned a client to me who was expected to lose all his vision within 3 months. Mr. Snider wanted to learn how to weave rugs on a floor loom while he still had some vision so he would be able to make and sell his rugs when his sight was gone. Mr. Snider soaked up my instruction. I taught him everything that would make him independent in this craft, including how to use up every bit of his material. I was glad that I could help him beat the clock on his blindness. However, his finished rugs did not sell well, and the Sales Department reported this to Mr. Ryan.

Mr. Ryan was blunt as he asked me whether I knew enough about weaving to teach it. "Yes," I told him. "I am sure I do and I know how to teach it to a person without sight, but I don't know much about what sells." Mr. Ryan quickly reacted by requesting his two blind rehabilitation workers, whose job it was to secure employment for the board's clients, to visit the buyers at a prominent department store in town and show them the rugs. They did this. The buyers assured them that the rugs were well made. However, they also noted that the rugs varied too much in size, color, width, and depth of borders (as a result of my teaching Mr. Snider not to waste anything). The buyers suggested using only primary-color cottons, making consistent four-inch fringe borders at both ends, and weaving each rug to conform to an exact length and width.

I explained the changes to Mr. Snider, who was intelligent and possessed grit. I told him I appreciated his gracious response to the changes. He always had displayed a stoic exterior, and our relationship was formal and businesslike. This expression of regret on my part (mostly an apology) for his need to plan differently actually brought more natural friendliness and warmth into our relationship, and it balanced out the exacting instruction

I had to give. Using friendly warmth promoted our connection in the occupation in which we were engaged, and it softened the hardships not only of his work but also of his condition. I learned from this to greatly soften my natural reserve, to demonstrate my friendliness willingly without retaliating to meet any stiffness I found in others.

The colors he used were tied in bundles so that he would not have to worry about errors; by now he was totally blind. And *voilà!* Mr. Snider's rugs sold rapidly after that. It cheered him, and I was introduced to that aspect of marketing for the first time. Many decades later the subject would resonate with occupational therapists as they would be required to understand how to match the goals of treatment with what reimbursement agencies would be willing to pay. This is different from selling material items that are not exactly in the province of occupational therapy, but recognizing the place of economics is important. The marketplace is a fundamental influence on all existence.

Helping Diane Show Her Mother "She Could Do It"

There were many memorable times with clients. Becoming blind after having vision is a cataclysmic event. Many a life becomes a disaster for a while until some balance is recovered. I was privileged to work with a very pretty high school senior, Diane, who had suddenly lost all her sight from a serious case of childhood diabetes. We shopped together so that she could learn to manage her money and plan a budget to gain greater independence. We talked a lot about her new experiences with blindness. She told me that the boys used to compete for dates with her but now no one asked her out. When we walked in the street together men and boys noticed her, then suddenly they would become aware of something in her gaze that caused them to freeze and simply stare.

However, Diane had an amazingly high emotional IQ. Despite her sadness she had decided to rise to the challenge of being blind. She was philosophical about her loss but also frustrated because she felt blocked by her family. Her mother in particular was overprotective and prevented her from exploring skills or joining groups she wanted to try. Yet her own temperament was such that she did not show outward anger or become depressed. Rather, she kept trying to change her family's attitude toward her blindness. She believed that she needed to bide her time. It pleased her family when, a few years later, she married a young man who had partial vision. They made each other happy.

A feature of the Board for Services to the Blind was that no client was ever considered discharged, because the condition of blindness implied that some additional services might be required throughout life. Therefore, even after she was married, Diane and I continued our visits for reviewing skills and learning tasks that related to her interests. One day, I invited her to my home for an afternoon visit. She told me the following story. During the previous week, her mother had come to visit her. Alone, Diane had baked blueberry muffins and was removing them from the oven when her mother arrived. She expressed surprise that Diane had developed so much ability. While they sat enjoying coffee and muffins, her mother exclaimed that they were the best muffins she had ever had. Then Diane related that in church that morning she felt the warmth of the sun stream in through the windows onto her hands. Her beautiful, radiant face displayed her happiness as she described the insight she experienced at the moment she became aware of the sun. "I have come to believe that everyone must have their special purpose for being born. I feel my purpose was to make those blueberry muffins to show my mother I could do it." Three weeks later, she suddenly died of a massive heart attack. She had had very delicate health but very sturdy beliefs and had achieved what she felt was important in her short life. I took comfort with the realization that Diane had lost her sight but never her inner vision of what she wanted and did accomplish.

Connecting Judy to the Community Across 50 Years

Another client I met in 1951 was a young woman, a few years younger than me, who was deaf and blind. Judy did see shadows and some colors on very clear days. Sitting close beside her, speaking distinctly and slowly into her right ear, I could communicate with her. She did not need a home teacher because she had graduated from the School for the Blind at the age of 20 and had many skills. Mr. Ryan referred her to me because he believed she needed community contacts. I made arrangements for her to attend a dance program at the local YWCA, and I took her there until she became comfortable going alone in a taxi. There she danced with a volunteer, a man who owned a clock factory, and he learned from her how much she wanted a job. He hired her and she enjoyed working for him for several years until his business closed.

Judy understood how to help herself and how to benefit from the help of others when the opportunity arose to speak up for herself. While I worked at the board, Judy and I remained in contact as I taught her salable crafts. During those times we also discussed options she could use when problems arose in her life. Even after I left the board, she and I continued communicating for a few decades but then lost touch. In early 1999, I was surprised to receive a letter from Judy renewing our contact. I offered to visit her at her home in a distant town. She lived alone and had held several jobs over the years; she told me that she had been in her current job for 19 years.

She now was totally blind, and her deafness had increased. I was pleased to find her looking very young for her 68 years, neat and composed in appearance and with naturally curly gray hair. Her greatest need continues to be to obtain regular social interaction. She spoke passionately of her fears that she would be alone for too many days in her apartment when she retires. She sees that her siblings are dying, and younger family members may be too busy for her.

During my visit I noticed a cassette player and reminded her that it could be useful to her. She had forgotten how to use it and thought it was broken because she had not realized that the pause button was down. Together we reviewed several plans for using the player, and I again enjoyed working on solutions with her. I observed that she read a weekly Braille copy of the *New York Times*. But those were mild pacifiers in the total picture of her need to feel connected with the outside world.

Judy made me aware of how acceptance of help from others can be full of compromise and irony. When someone volunteers to help Judy shop for groceries, for example, her decisions often were overridden. The helper would tell her to wait for the article to go on sale, or buy a cheaper substitute she did not want, or even questioned her need for an item—especially if the helper did not like it. The recitation of her lament sounded like good material for a stand-up comic, and it made me want to laugh despite the sadness of the story.

Several months later when I telephoned to schedule another visit, I noted how easy she made it for me to communicate with her. I spoke in short, clear sentences. She repeated them. If she heard me incorrectly, I would say no and repeat what I said. If she heard me correctly, I went on. She exclaimed her gratefulness for my call and did not mention the length of time I had let go by before calling her again. I complimented her on a letter she sent me, and she reminded me that she had written it on the same typewriter that I had helped her obtain almost 50 years before. She told me that on the date I proposed to visit her that she might be leaving for camp in another state. This was the same camp I had enrolled her in nearly a half-century before. Her perky responses lacked self-pity. Judy often observed poignantly the contrast between what normal people called "problems" and her unrelenting ones. She would add, wryly, that life gave her handicaps while normal people seemed intent on creating their own.

Judy remembered and reminded me about the contacts, lasting adaptations, arrangements, and special events we had worked out together. When I told her I had forgotten, she laughed and said, "I remember because they were important to me." Having the opportunity to respond to Judy at different stages in her life also made me realize that it is easier to make arrangements to take people shopping, get them to medical appointments, and meet the other concrete needs of people with disabilities than it is to meet the deeper human need for relief from loneliness and isolation. Nonetheless, Judy impressed on me the relevance and the long-standing worthwhile results that an occupational therapy approach accomplishes with people with disabilities.

In 2001, Judy retired. Just as she feared, her contacts with others outside of her family became almost nonexistent. When I visited her, she seemed to have aged radically. I sought contact with the state's Board of Education and Services for the Blind to find out what assistance might be available to her. People from the board and from other associations familiar to her visited to explain that federal funds had been put aside for her to use to pay helpers for well-defined duties for a given number of hours each week. Although Judy was not thriving by being alone so much, she refused the funds.

Up to now, Judy had always had family members to take her to appointments, to fix equipment that had broken in her apartment, or to handle her financial matters. Sometimes volunteers helped by visiting her. However, she had never seen herself as a manager who might hire assistance. The proposition the board made seemed unreasonable. For one thing, the amount seemed excessive to her—possibly more than she herself had ever earned. The offer seemed to shock her sensibilities. It took time to find ways for her to view matters differently for her benefit, and perhaps her family helped in this. My intention was to try to understand what I could do.

I assumed the role of advocate and began to call people regularly at the Board of Education and Services for the Blind to inquire about the status of services for Judy. Advocacy required persistent telephone calls to many people; many of those I had started at first to call retired during the few years that I continued. I finally sent letters to the director of services at the board, the Connecticut attorney general, and local and federal representatives. Resolution of several mishaps had to occur before there were results. Eventually, my quest for the release and payment of adequate funds for the skilled visitor was realized in March 2004. A person, knowledgeable about the issues of people who are deaf and blind, visits with Judy once a month. It is only a beginning of what Judy requires, and the advocacy needs to continue. However, even this little bit of regular visiting seemed to brighten her appearance.

I saw that Judy could speak up for herself when she required a job, but self-advocacy was harder for her when it came to nurturing friendships or obtaining services. Her early situation of having parental protection and many siblings to help her prevented her and those around her from becoming aware that this could not last. She became angry with me when I suggested that she take cookies to a neighbor she wanted to meet. She was capable of doing it; she just did not seem to feel comfortable about it. Or she forbade me to ask a sighted member of her family to help advocate for her at a social agency. I explained to her that she needs to tell her guides when she is at a social function to introduce her to at least four other people with whom she can shake hands. She liked this when I did it with her at a function.

Judy believes that others in the community should come forward to help her of their own accord and that her blindness is too large a handicap for her to override for obtaining most normal desires. She would not allow discussion that I might have with her on proactive activity on her part.

The family of a child born with blindness must provide early training for greater self-reliance in social matters, and Judy's family neglected to attend to that part of her education in her childhood years. It also is clear that Judy rises above her rage, her despair, and her unfulfilled yearnings by maintaining a high standard in chosen areas. Her home is always neat, as is her grooming, her organization of matters such as shopping for food, and putting away personal supplies. She attends church regularly, remembers important dates and details about relatives and friends, writes thank you notes, and stays as much as possible in touch with changes in the world. She has a good sense of humor, incredible empathy for other people's calamities, and always demonstrates a special dignity. Those attributes promote respect and admiration for her. Judy knows what she wants, and, when given the opportunity, she has made good decisions. She is greatly cheered up when she can look forward to an outing, and there is a start of this for her now. Her assigned visitor from the board has shared with me that she also has noticed a more mellow and upbeat attitude in Judy.

It was with a feeling of great glee that I finally heard from her visitor in November 2004 that she has achieved further assurance that she may increase her visits to take Judy out twice a month. It occurred very naturally—Judy had to sign a paper at the time of each visit and thus learned that the visit was being reimbursed. Because the money did not pass through Judy, it appears to be acceptable to her. Advocacy is the way to go!

I happened at the time to be in an exercise group with Joan, the skilled worker assigned by the Board of Education and Services for the Blind. She knew about my special concern for Judy, and she sent me excerpts of some of her visit reports. During the first year, her visits were for shopping, the hairdresser, bingo at a senior center, and having lunch out. But more interesting events developed. Judy's membership in a knitting group at the senior center greatly enhanced her life.

JULY 2005

Dear Mildred,

Saw Judy yesterday, Thursday. Went to Needleworks [knitting] at Senior Center. Met Margaret and Mary who live at Rabnud, apartment building for seniors. Rabnud holds knitting classes also on Monday mornings. Red Cross supplies yarn and needles. Margaret encouraged Judy to come. Judy would like to. Note: Margaret's granddaughter is deaf, so she learned sign language 30 years ago! A very sociable day!

Joan

[Unfortunately, there was no one to take Judy on Monday, so this did not work out.]

AUGUST 2005

Was really pleased by yesterday's activities with Judy! In knitting group, Judy was given 3 skeins of worsted. And coordinator of group gave me print pattern for child's hat. I put pattern into Braille and will mail it on Saturday after buying her a pair of size 8 needles. Judy seems pleased that this project will occupy her time, and the hats are sent to poor children in Europe. A mitzvah for all?!

SEPTEMBER 2005

Writing with more good news and an interesting philosophical comment from Judy, both about her knitting. She brought the almost finished child's hat to the knitting/crochet group: People praised and complimented her often! She thanked the women but later, out in the car, commented that sighted people often are amazed by what blind people can accomplish. What happens now? Mary, one of the knitters, will finish off the last 9 stitches and sew the seam. Judy left the group with empty needles and the request for another hat. They have also asked her to make hat and scarf sets for young children. I will look for a much lighter weight yarn for her.

OCTOBER 2005

After 3 or 3¹/₂ hours, we both run out of energy. Grocery shopping takes time; the background voices make it harder to hear!...Knitting group: a blessing for Judy. Mary P., the woman who sews the seam, took the time to talk with her yesterday. Seems many women, like Judy, had parents who emigrated from Italy. Judy misses the convenience of having someone shop for her weekly. But when I mentioned asking the city's senior center if they had a Friendly Shopper program, she hesitated. I'll look into it.
[Judy later declined the help.]

FEBRUARY 2006

Two weeks ago, at lunch, Judy wanted to talk with Mary, a neighbor, about a power outage that occurred during heavy rain. Yesterday, one of the Bingo players—with whom we often shared a table—came to meet Judy to learn how she was doing. There's a lot more interaction since the knitting group. Thank God! I talked with her about the national deaf–blind convention in June. She still does not want to go. The cost for the delegates is quite steep, and her energy level is less than what it used to be.

MARCH 2006

Wanted to send some news of my day spent with Judy. A good day! We met at 1:30 p.m. for a family concert: Taubl Family from New Hampshire. Seven children, ages 10 to 21 who are all accomplished musicians on string instruments. Most of the children introduced the selections. I later learned that Judy could not hear what was spoken or sung; she could hear the instrumental pieces. I asked if she would rather not go next year because she misses "chunks." She said she wants to go again because last year (mandolin concert) and this year brought music she's never heard before! Nice to hear that! I see Judy again in 2 weeks for lunch, haircut, and groceries.

APRIL 2006
Two weeks ago, Judy told me that she and her niece talked about a concert at her church performed on string instruments by a family of 7 children. I had gone with Judy to this concert when it had been given at a Senior Center. This gave Judy a topic for conversation.

MAY 2006
Worked with Judy yesterday. Wanted to share two anecdotes. At the town's Health Fair for seniors, Judy spoke with a representative of a speech and hearing center. They told her they would accept her Dr.'s note saying Medicare should pay, and they accept Medicare for evaluations. But Judy's not convinced Medicare will pay the whole fee. And because they cannot tell her the cause of her deafness, she will not make an appointment. ... Also, a member of the knitting group is buying and donating yarn to the Rabnud apartment complex for some time because the Red Cross has not come to bring yarn for some time. This member also brought three skeins for Judy in the Thursday group as well. Kind woman!

Those anecdotal reports illustrate how profoundly the skill of knitting has opened important doors for Judy; she had something purposeful to do when alone, people to relate to, and some small broadening of relationships in her neighborhood. However, Judy frequently rejected opportunities for the possibility of additional escorts, for benefits that might accrue to her from hearing tests, or for grant assistance that could help relieve her isolation. She requires an advocate by her side to carefully explain what is being offered to her. The board-assigned skilled worker is not trained to do this; what Joan could offer is some relief from isolation, provide for a dependable schedule of at least monthly outings, and offer the possibility that, like the sunshine appearance of the knitting group, some other opportunity might present itself in which Judy can become absorbed.

Losing Skilled Supervision for the First Time

When Mr. Ryan was forced to retire at the age of 70, I spent some time trying to accept the new director. He was unsuited for the position, incompetent and indifferent to the population he served. I resigned from the agency. That new director also resigned 5 years later when the Association of Blind Persons (ABP) rose up against him and demanded his dismissal, the first of many ethical issues I was to witness in my work.

Perhaps ABP's membership also remembered Mr. Ryan's fairness and compassion. With quiet good humor and endless wisdom, he conveyed to each one a sense of his or her personal worth. From his example, people who were blind learned how they should expect to be treated. It was a testimony to him when they demonstrated in a united complaint against an unworthy director and won.

Mr. Ryan lacked defensiveness or a need to worry about protecting himself. He exuded an uncomplicated trust in others, attending with interest to what others had to say and directing this with ease. He seemed indifferent to status, and he was greatly revered by those who knew him. Mr. Ryan had been a strong leader and a wonderful guide; he had been patient and kind and always forthright. He taught me standards as he focused on the love and value of the work he did and the people he served. I never have found a rival to his greatness as a principled human being.

CLOSENESS, CONNECTION, AND OBJECTIVITY

Until the middle of the 20th century, it was widely accepted that people in psychiatric hospitals were committed for life. It is interesting that, in the early part of the century, many state psychiatric hospitals were built on sites with exquisite natural vistas, often on a body of water (Tomes, 1994). Sometimes those committed even were brought by boat to the psychiatric hospital. In the early days, patients were "sent down the river," never to return. A change in thinking in the 1950s and 1960s led to a shift in understanding: After an extended period of hospitalization, sometimes years, and with appropriate pharmaceutical treatment, a person with mental illness could possibly be discharged to the community (Padilla, 2005a; Torrey, 1997).

I felt drawn to working in mental health, because it had become clear to me that there is a psychosocial component, an emotional aspect, to every disability. I saw this when I worked with people who were blind. I believed that by working in what is now called *behavioral health,* I would recapture the great feeling of pleasure in learning and accomplishment that I had had working with those who were blind.

Coming to Undercliff Hospital

For the rest of the 1950s I worked at the Undercliff Hospital in Meriden, Connecticut. Undercliff was a tuberculosis sanitarium that had been converted to a psychiatric facility. The staff had been "converted," too: The tuberculosis specialists had to become psychiatrists overnight, and the rest of the employees had to learn new skills as well. We all learned together. By that time I had more confidence as I met the new, and sometimes ludicrous, circumstances.

The hospital's program was for people who were on the road to mental health recovery but needed more recuperation time to acquire skills and to set goals for themselves. Patients were not expected to be in an acute state of illness and were selected by recommendation from the three larger state psychiatric hospitals. With little experience in understanding people with psychiatric illnesses, Undercliff's physicians lacked the skill to interview with insight, and selections were not always made with adequate judgment. The physicians often based their choices on the appearance of the people recommended for transfer but slowly learned that this method was inadequate. Sometimes patients required more recovery time in the original facility and were not ready for our programs. This affected the availability of placements, as some patients needed to remain longer than originally planned.

Occupational therapy was an important component of treatment at Undercliff. Many of the people admitted could benefit from learning the demanding and purposeful crafts taught there. Completion of a craft item often was a source of pride for the patients, especially when they uncovered new talents or skills. Patients assigned to the occupational therapy clinic learned silk screening; metal etching; manual typesetting and printing on upright presses; or leatherwork, which consisted of cutting the pieces of a project, like a purse, from large pieces of cowhide (the kits generally available today were not on the market then). Adele Caudle, OTR/L, was the supervisor of the department and always demonstrated great flexibility, understanding, and resourcefulness. She was a great teacher, and we became lifelong friends.

More important, the substance of good treatment was stressed. The therapist worked individually to adapt activities to each person's aptitudes and needs. The activities chosen were those that promote concentration and require the organizing actions of planning, using judgment, and making decisions, because those skills are diminished in mental illness.

Overcoming Despair With Problem Solving

One elderly patient assigned to me was Ms. Cowry, a former ballerina who had been diagnosed with a psychotic depression. She had drawing talent and asked me to show her how to enamel on copper. Enameling requires steady hands, and because her hands had a tremor, we had to solve the problem of how to adapt the task for her. I saw how her cleverness, artistry, and creativity in accomplishment gave her much pleasure. Among several items she created was an exquisite picture of a bouquet of irises on a 2-inch copper disk. She dropped small gobs of color and, using a very fine tipped brush, her left hand stabilizing her carefully positioned right, she made a dark outline around the color and created an iris. This became a pin as I soldered a pin-back and a copper loop on the back so that the disk could be a pendant as well. I was permitted to buy this from her for a fair amount, much to her delight, and it always elicited praise from others when my mother wore the pin. Ms. Cowry demonstrated courage and elegance as she worked hard to push away the clouds of despair and chose to concentrate on the problems her pin designs presented. She succeeded.

Sharing Was Shakespearean Actor's Medicine

Another patient was a Shakespearean actor who had appeared on Broadway. We formed a poetry group, and he interpreted Shakespeare's sonnets during many of the sessions. All the group members watched and listened to him with rapt attention. I learned never to underestimate the hunger all people have for the beauty found in the arts. I scurried about to find poems with dialogue when I noticed the men often wanted to read the female voices and the women would volunteer for the male voices. I responded to the significance of it without understanding it fully at the time. "The Death of the Hired Man" by Robert Frost (Untermeyer, 1971) was a favorite with this group. I was being introduced to the benefits of group participation as people interacted and learned from each other. It would become a lasting interest for me throughout my professional life. And the Shakespearean actor became my first instructor. I still can feel the intensity of his love of the arts, his talent, and his wish to share it with everyone despite his personal difficulties. Giving was his medicine.

Creating Art and Good Outcomes

The arts hold a very strong place in mental health. The act of creating and producing requires focus and concentration, even if only a minimal amount of these qualities can be forthcoming at first. In the very act of initiating a production, anxieties can be reduced, if only for a short time. Creating artwork often allows patients to express emotional stress in a nonconfrontational way, leading to potentially meaningful verbalization.

At Undercliff, I worked every day with patients who would stay for a year or more. Because hospitalization was prolonged, it would have been easy to become overly involved with patients. That was my opportunity to learn how to permit necessary closeness and connection yet preserve the objectivity required in a therapeutic relationship. It brought home my need to consider and build my own understanding of how to behave compassionately with a person to establish and honor both sets of boundaries. Fortunately, there were sympathetic staff members to talk with and good supervisory counseling. My own reflective processes, learned earlier, helped me learn to question myself first before acting.

I saw good outcomes at the discharge of patients: Many sought more education, a better place to live, or new employment. I developed a great interest in behavioral health practice during my stay of almost 5 years at Undercliff. I left that full-time position when my second child was born in 1960.

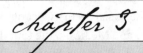

THE 1960S:
BALANCING MOTHERHOOD AND WORK

NEW DIRECTIONS IN OCCUPATIONAL THERAPY

Confronting Change

In the 1960s, my career interests were suspended so that I could focus on my children. My third child was born in this decade. For many Americans, it was a time to confront traditional values and beliefs about science, politics, and civil rights. I was not prepared for the gradual disappearance of the professional world I had known. Under the comforting blanket of 1950s contentment, when it seemed nothing would ever change, I failed to hear the rumblings of suppressed needs and bolder demands. In general, there remained a resistance to examining the status quo.

The 1960s unfolded with many changing events! Important discoveries occurred. Among other milestones was the new polio vaccine. That disease had been a scourge for a quarter-century, but it also provided the training ground for treatment of physical disabilities. Improved psychiatric drugs helped squash the notion that entering a mental hospital was a sentence for life.

The great courage expressed by leaders in the civil rights movement may well have inspired the push for many diverse groups to gather their strength and move on their own struggle to right the wrongs that existed for them. "Tell it like it is" became the mainstream message of many groups: racial minorities, union workers, gay men or lesbians, and feminists. Family life was stripped of its idealized storefront window. Donna Reed went down the tubes, and Father didn't know best anymore (Padilla, 2005b). No, say it isn't so!

At the same time, a new sense of responsibility to be committed to change was heard in President John F. Kennedy's 1961 rallying cry, "ask not what your country can do for you—ask what you can do for your country." With the Social Security Act of 1965, President Lyndon B. Johnson created Medicare and Medicaid, the foundations of his Great Society programs, which helped Americans become aware of the citizens previously kept hidden from sight. The needs of those with disabilities marked the decade and created a new urgency for the helping arts and sciences, among them occupational therapy. Stepping out into space as our astronauts did encouraged others to aspire to nobler dreams and possibilities in the cosmos and in whatever realm they occupied. That spirit was reflected in the therapies as new approaches in intervention emerged.

The new freedom exposed the suppressed emotions and secret desires that were thought to block healthy behavior. Young people would express this new freedom through music and poetry in a tidal wave of events from Woodstock to San Francisco. A keen sense of daring to be different, a new kind of individualism leveled the distance between the haves and the have-nots. All of the professions responded to those changes with a tolerance for differences in behavior and appearances, and that affected occupational therapy as well. The period was a precursor to the legislative changes that would come in the next decade to meet the special needs of the disabled population. Emphasis on education and a more accessible environment were initiated. And the increasingly unpopular Vietnam War led to uneasiness that was followed by cynicism about our leaders and further emboldened the public to question the establishment.

Discovering New Ideas in Occupational Therapy

Catching the mood, new directions emerged during the 1960s in the American Occupational Therapy Association (AOTA). A gifted guide and prolific writer, Wilma L. West (1916–1996), was president of AOTA from 1961 to 1964 (AOTA, 1985b). As she introduced her vision for the profession in many of her writings and speeches (Cox & West, 1982; West, 1958, 1976, 1982, 1992), she championed advanced education, advocated for graduate programs for occupational therapists, and insisted that research was vital for proving the effectiveness of the profession (and AOTA's *Centennial Vision* echoes these same goals today; AOTA, 2007; Brachtesende, 2007). Later, Ms. West was instrumental in establishing the American Occupational Therapy Foundation (ATOF), which encouraged research. During her 1972–1982 term as president of AOTF, she underwrote the hiring of the first librarian to classify and organize its collection of resources, journals, and books. The current librarian (recently retired), Mary Binderman, said West moved with purpose on many of her convictions for occupational therapy: "A main factor was her belief that occupational therapy had a knowledge base, which it needed to expand and to maintain with the assistance of the library" (M. Binderman, personal communication, August 8, 2007). West was an early proponent of moving occupational therapy from the hospital to the community. She foresaw that a person's environment is a strong influence to be considered in the treatment plan. Wilma West was ahead of her time, and several decades passed before occupational therapy would actualize the far-reaching accomplishments she had in mind and today we take for granted (Foto, 1997; Gillette, 1998; West, 1989, 1990).

A. Jean Ayres, PhD, entered the field in the mid-1940s when she began to treat children and adults with neurological disorders (Ayres, 1972). Her treatments were traditional, but her observations led her to obtain advanced coursework in brain physiology. In the late 1950s and throughout the 1960s, Dr. Ayres researched and wrote about learning as she developed her theories about sensory integration disorders. Her legacy to the practice of occupational therapy is her vast work and writing on sensory integration treatment and interventions (Ayres, 1979; Ayres, Erwin, & Mailloux, 2004; Ayres, Henderson, Llorens, Gilfoyle, Myers, & Prevel, 1974). Occupational therapists began to use her work in schools, and today sensory integration therapy is an essential part of many school programs and pediatric clinics.

The work in group dynamics and in the new kinds of groups that developed in the 1960s began to enthrall me, although I had received no training for it. Three occupational therapists, Gail Fidler, OTR; Lela Llorens, OTR; and Anne Mosey, OTR, began to document the work that was their legacy to the profession (Fidler & Fidler, 1964; Llorens, 1976; Mosey, 1973). Others soon took up the study that would influence occupational therapy groups. In the second edition of *Group Dynamics in Occupational Therapy* (1998), Marilyn Cole refers to their contributions. Art, music, dance, and horticulture—formerly used exclusively by occupational therapists—became independent areas of therapy, although at the time they were usually under the aegis of occupational therapy departments. There would be more changes as practitioners grew in independence.

Occupational therapy positions were plentiful in hospitals and long-term-care facilities. Government funding was available because occupational therapy was considered part of the health care package. It was assumed that occupational therapy already had proven itself as a valuable adjunct to medicine.

Staying Connected to My Work

I left the psychiatric hospital in 1960 to devote time to my children, but I still wanted to work 8 or 10 hours a week. At the time, however, anything less than full-time employment generally was not available, per diem work had not been invented, and most mothers were not encouraged to work outside the home. In my search for an hourly position, I discovered the nursing homes and regional agencies for children and adults with mental retardation. Most of the facilities were dismal, and the establishment did not even deem it necessary to disguise the bluntly custodial care offered to the residents. I knew I could not provide worthwhile service in so few hours in those places, even if they would consider hiring me.

Eventually, I found a part-time position in a retirement facility for Catholic nuns. In 1960, the federal minimum wage was $1 an hour, and it was just $1.70 by the end of the decade. My wages were comparable to 21st-century pay scales: The $5 per hour I earned was the equivalent of about $26 per hour today. Although I was keeping my hand in occupational therapy, I was isolated from my peers even as I was aware that exciting changes were taking place. I struggled with the now-familiar tension of wanting to be a full-time mother and a full-time professional.

At the time, the best way to stay in touch was to attend meetings of my professional state organization, the Connecticut Occupational Therapy Association (ConnOTA). I depended on the group for information and advocacy about legislation to protect my practice and my profession. ConnOTA also was an important source of lasting relationships in my life. I remember the especially effective presidency of Barbara (Bobby) Steward. We eventually attended workshops together, and our friendship grew.

Bobby Steward became a professor in the occupational therapy program at Quinnipiac College (now University) and, as she experimented with the newer therapies, she shared her knowledge with me. She was a great source of support later when I needed encouragement to present the workshops I had developed on my group model. One special presentation she reviewed with me was for California's Atascadero State Hospital in 1991 and again in 1992. I wanted to emphasize the effects of activities on the central nervous system and how that information can be used in planning group treatment. Atascadero State is a huge hospital for people charged with crimes and diagnosed with mental illness. Because I felt well-prepared, I enjoyed the experience.

There always was a great reciprocity in friendships with occupational therapists in ConnOTA. That is an important reason for membership in one's professional organization. I remember the extraordinary helpfulness of Lois Carlson, OTR/L, CHT, when I served as an interim president in ConnOTA in the 1980s. She took the assignment of an important project no one else wanted, and it was a success. She extended herself in other ways. She eventually became the first recipient in 1992 of the Healthsouth Rehabilitation Award for Clinical Excellence.

Indeed in the 1960s, 1970s, and early 1980s, occupational therapists championed the initiation of new programs in Connecticut that were to strengthen the profession. Janet Small developed the COTA (Certified Occupational Therapy Assistant) program. Mary Fiorentino, director of a pediatric program, wrote widely on the influence of primitive reflexes on motor development (1963, 1974, 1981). Important national issues like licensure, reimbursement, and CEUs (continuing education units) for occupational therapists were instituted earlier in Connecticut than in many other states.

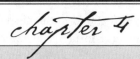

THE 1970S:
PHYSICAL DISABILITIES AND MENTAL HEALTH

A DIFFERENT VISION FOR PATIENT CARE

The changes in occupational therapy treatment that began in the 1960s were consolidated in the 1970s. When I returned to work full time at Cedarcrest Hospital, a state hospital for physical disabilities, activities with small woodworking tools or wooden frames for hand weaving might be used. But therapeutic use of arts and crafts came under scrutiny as clinics began to consider leatherwork, hand-setting of type, and metal etching as expendable luxuries. A more practical approach was to focus on self-care and training in work skills for productivity in the home and out of it, such as dressing and cooking. I began to attend workshops involving neuroscience in the treatment in physical and mental trauma. Occupational therapists also used hands-on manipulation of muscles or explored how learning in the damaged brain could be improved with the new therapeutic interventions (Fiorentino, 1974). I was not prepared for the changes, despite my growing awareness and curiosity.

The vision grew that people who had been hospitalized or institutionalized might be treated in the community, and in the 1970s the treatment and discharge pace in hospitals intensified (Mace & Rabins, 1981; Torrey, 1997). Federal and state legislation (U.S. Department of Justice, 2005) mandated that children with learning disabilities, physical disabilities, and developmental disabilities receive education and then publicly funded job training in what were then called *sheltered workshops*. In the ensuing decades, those foundational laws would be enhanced into firmer and more guarantees of rights for people with disabilities through the Americans with Disabilities Act of 1990 and the Individuals with Disabilities Education Act Amendments of 1997.

By the mid-1970s, hospitals began planning discharge at the time of admission. Only the very sick stayed in the hospital; short-term treatment of a few weeks or months was considered adequate for those for whom an earlier recovery could be anticipated. In health care, occupational therapy was acknowledged as tremendously viable, respected, and essential. Occupational therapists continued to hold important leadership roles in mental health care.

Returning to a Vibrant Profession

As my children were growing up, I was glad that I had given my time to their early years. By 1970, however, when I wanted to return to full-time work, I did not have many choices. I was not ready for work in a long-term-care setting, and the application of occupational therapy in school systems was not as widely developed as it is today. A few occupational therapists had private practices, but that was not an option I would consider because it seemed to lack security. However, occupational therapy had become a vibrant profession, with new vocabularies, theories and techniques, clinical tools, aspirations, and popular leaders who reflected the general dynamism of the decade.

A. Jean Ayres's (1972) theories and research on sensory integration bristled in the air, bringing exciting new energy that influenced treatment for children and adults alike. Earlier retreats for state and corporate employees called *encounter groups* that began in the 1960s would influence the therapeutic groups conducted with patients (Lowen, 1966). Those employee retreats consisted of both somber and joyous forays into sharing feelings and connecting with other members of one's own and other disciplines, and they foreshadowed the group process that soon became part of many occupational therapy curricula. The need for more expertise in group therapy was being recognized.

In the early 1970s, Lorna Jean King, OTR/L (1974), introduced her work with groups of people with schizophrenia. That practice drew on her knowledge of neurology and sensory integration.

Continuing education workshops were not as prevalent as they are today, but the number was growing. The early workshops I attended in occupational therapy emphasized the structure of the central nervous system and its relationship to new facilitation methods for the treatment of physical disabilities and perceptual problems that occurred in learning disorders and as a result of brain trauma.

MOVING FROM PASSIVE PATIENT TO CONNECTED CLIENT

I was hired as a full-time staff therapist in 1970 at Cedarcrest, a Connecticut state hospital for people with chronic physical disabilities. Cedarcrest had two facilities on its grounds: a tuberculosis sanitarium that was being shut down and a larger hospital building that admitted patients with physical trauma, both chronic and acute.

Jane Olsen, OTR, supervised the Cedarcrest occupational therapy clinic. She embodied confidence with her competence and love for her work. She used an assortment of minor crafts and purposeful activities to mobilize the paralyzed limbs of stroke patients, and she taught adaptive working techniques to people who had been in accidents or who had lost limbs and needed to learn to use prostheses. Her other patients included those with brain injury, palsy, arthritis, or other debilitating conditions acquired at birth or through trauma.

The occupational therapist was expected to provide an assessment relevant to the referral that analyzed the patient's abilities and needs. From this assessment, the therapist created the sequence of treatment and goals for the patient. The patient's role was a passive one so far, and the label *patient* seemed appropriate.

Gradual changes began in the 1970s, and I had the following experience. Mary, a client whose stroke had resulted in weakness in her left arm and left leg, had been referred by her doctor to occupational therapy for retraining in activities of daily living (ADLs). I assessed her status and developed a treatment plan without much collaboration with her, as was the usual routine.

One day I could not find her on the ward and asked the nurse where she might be. The nurse told me that she believed Mary was not interested in my program; perhaps she was giving me this message by her absence. The nurse suggested that my attitude might need modification. Occupational therapy had a mission, but Mary's expectation for herself had to be understood as well. This was a criticism I needed. I had to institute discussion and collaboration, and I needed a deeper understanding of others' needs, including Mary's need to be in control of her choices.

Pushing too earnestly, I would learn, imposes on the client the therapist's ambitions instead of imposing on the therapist an appreciation of the client's wishes and requirements. I became aware that my idea of independence—

or any goal—might not match the client's wishes. What to me might seem a practical way of looking at life can be an arrogant assumption seen through the client's eyes.

Thirty years ago, very few sick people questioned or evaluated the path of their treatment. What was ordered usually was obediently followed. Slowly, that attitude changed. In the 21st century, participation in one's own health and the position of self-advocacy, if not universally practiced, are readily accepted. That significant shift toward self-determination was fueled externally by the emerging culture of individualism that began in the 1960s and that caused the setting of treatment goals to become collaborative and client centered, rather than unilateral (Law, 1998). Clients need to express their own wishes for themselves and to question the therapeutic and medical decisions made for them.

Overwhelmed by the changes in practice in the early 1970s, I became a workshop addict; one year I attended 30, most of them consisting of 2 days of instruction. At that time, the state was enthusiastic about continuing education, and my employer covered the expense and gave me time to attend the training.

The continuing education workshops presented by Josephine C. Moore, OTR, PhD, FAOTA, were my favorites. Dr. Moore taught gross anatomy in the medical school at South Dakota State University, and she presented lectures on the central nervous system to occupational therapists and other professionals throughout the country. In addition to her scientific and teaching expertise, she has a great artistic talent. As she spoke, she illustrated her subject by drawing on the blackboard the complex nervous system. For the next 20 years, I attended many of her workshops. One time I asked Dr. Moore to read excerpts from my writings that involved the use of physiological principles I applied to practice. I wanted to be certain that I was correctly using what I had learned. I am extremely grateful and fortunate that she generously extended this kindness to me for two of my early books.

I finally heard A. Jean Ayres, the leader in learning disability research in the world of occupational therapy, speak in 1970 when she came to Connecticut to offer a workshop. She introduced sensory integration theory, which synthesized the burgeoning field of visual–motor–perceptual theories for explaining how the brain learns and how to apply that understanding in the treatment of learning disabilities. Dr. Ayres began her lecture straightaway as though she were continuing a conversation started just moments before. There were no welcoming remarks, jokes, or other pleasantries that so many use as ice breakers. She was serious and all-business, and the audience hung on her every word. Several years later, when I viewed videotapes that showed her interactions with young clients, she was revealed as gentle and playful—an expert therapist.

As much as possible I integrated the increased knowledge into my work at Cedarcrest. The medical administration encouraged the use of new ideas and techniques in the clinic. Our department reported patients' progress in documentation kept in the medical records and at weekly medical interdisciplinary staff meetings. That seemed to assure the managing medical staff that we were doing our job.

About two years into my employment at Cedarcrest, Jane Olson was diagnosed with cancer. It was most distressing to me to observe her valiant struggle as she sought to maintain her dignity and privacy during her treatment. She stayed in her position as long as she could, and during her many absences, I was reluctant to move in on her turf to make any changes. One physician who was very interested in occupational therapy chided me, "How will anyone know, Mildred, if you can lead if you are walking behind Jane and not a few paces ahead when she is not here?" Nevertheless, I would not preempt her, and I hoped she would recover. She did not live, however, and the memory of her courageous struggle remains poignant to me.

After Jane's death, I was appointed supervisor of the Occupational Therapy Department. My staff consisted of one occupational therapist and one certified occupational therapist assistant (COTA), Ignea Leahy, who also was a personal friend. I had urged her to undertake COTA training because I knew she had special gifts for the work. The setting within my department was harmonious and ideal for experimenting with the new learning I was acquiring.

Proving Value in Occupational Therapy

However, the visiting physiatrist, as a consulting physician in physical medicine, conducted the weekly medical team meetings at Cedarcrest and seemed to give scant attention to our reports. His professional orientation likely led him to favor the goals of walking, a physical therapy treatment area, and talking, a speech therapy treatment area, over the goals for functional outcomes that our occupational therapy department emphasized. That aroused a competitive urge in our department to show that demonstrable function was possible even in a person who could not walk or talk. We were triumphant one day when one such patient, Sally, was discharged home, leaving in a wheelchair that was pushed by her caring husband. This is her story.

Our department staff had met with Sally's husband many times, openly discussing all the issues that had troubled him, from self-care and homemaking to social and personal issues. Sally, who was in her 40s, had had a severe stroke that affected her right dominant side, resulting in aphasia. She could not speak and displayed difficulty in understanding the speech of others, but she could sing a little. During her hospital stay, she never regained useful strength in her right arm and leg. We treated her for months, and she became independent in performing self-care. With minimum to moderate assistance, she achieved a good skill level in homemaking that we expected could improve with practice. She had worked hard to adapt to her short-term memory losses and easy distractibility. She could cook a simple meal, clean up, and do laundry, and she had learned how to use her family's help. Sally could not walk or talk—those were areas of emphasis for the physiatrist—but she displayed moderate success in those areas that had given her satisfaction and status before her illness, areas that she and her family thought important. Despite the physical losses, there was such great earnestness in Sally's efforts and those of her family that 35 years later the memory of her achievements inspires a transcendent joy in me.

There were always occasions when we had to work hard to inform and educate medical staff. Others encouraged us: Karoline Ascher was a staff physician who appreciated and supported our work. When she toured our department with visitors, I remember her using a sweeping, dramatic gesture that enveloped our entire clinic saying, "Here in occupational therapy, their assessments and results of therapy predict what we can expect from the patients during treatment and when they are discharged."

Recreational therapy was not a part of the hospital's program, although it was needed, and I frequently explained that our department could not provide "busy work" when a referral came with an order to keep a person "occupied." What we could do had to be described and explained continuously, so that all staff would understand the areas of our responsibility. When treatment requests were necessary, our small staff tried to comply by staggering treatment times to be less frequent but more comprehensive in covering the population. Positions were frequently frozen in the early 1970s. To get another therapist was not a priority with the managing medical staff—very much like today's conditions!

I emphasized facilitating communication among staff members in my department. At the time, each hospital created its own assessments. In keeping with the new approaches I was learning, I developed working evaluations that assessed ADLs and measured muscle strength. The staff was too small to work only with assigned patients; each of us had to be able to treat anyone ready to come to the clinic. I designed a worksheet of activities appropriate for any patient with neurological impairments. It included simpler to more difficult tasks that were congruent with the skills required by a patient who needed to gain functional independence. On any given day, the therapist could withdraw the sheet from a patient's folder, read the comments on past performance, and have a sense of what to pursue next. A continuity of progressive treatment was possible. My department seemed to be a busy, useful, and cheerful place.

Developing Client Groups

Marcia Donofrio, a registered physical therapist, introduced much sparkle into the rehabilitation program at Cedarcrest. She joined the physical therapy department during my time as the occupational therapy supervisor. She was a recent graduate who brought new vigor to her department. She suggested that we conduct a group together using exercise and discussion. Later, she suggested that we develop a home care program booklet for stroke patients to take with them upon discharge. The booklet had an introduction, our mantra of self-acceptance, our group exercises, and reminders for the functional tasks that are stressed in occupational therapy—such as self-care, brace care, homemaking skills, and leisure activities.

Very soon, she became disenchanted with her peers in physical therapy because they resisted all new learning. She wanted to transfer to my department and, much to my surprise, requested that the state health department arrange this. The department refused, stating that her training did not include a psychiatric affiliation, which in the department's opinion made all the difference between our disciplines. The department could not approve her request to be a therapist in an occupational therapy clinic! However, we realized that we could still enjoy working together, and we did.

It is obvious that the psychiatric affiliation was considered a huge plus for a therapist. During the psychiatric affiliation, the student can develop the understanding and the compassion required to help a client re-establish relationships that are upset whenever a disability is acquired. Often, it is the internal relationship the disabled person has that requires the most help, so it is important for the student to be introduced to psychosocial aspects of all disabling experiences. Marcia was an excellent therapist, and she recognized this. Good outcomes occurred as we worked together.

A compelling reason for sustaining our use of groups occurred one day when all of our group members were sitting in a circle with Marcia and me as we were about to begin the session. Suddenly, a new member looked around and burst into tears, "I don't want to be in a room with a bunch of cripples!" She fled the clinic. A bewildered silence followed that was broken by another member, "Now I know how far I've come. That was me 3 months ago." This was a seminal moment as I recognized the benefits that members bring to each other. This was the beginning of my passion to develop meaningful group sessions in the hospital. Groups would allow members to share with each other, and they would increase the practitioners' understanding through behavioral observation. I learned about conducting groups by observing the outcomes of our sessions. After each session, Marcia and I analyzed what worked and what did not. Working with Marcia was a joyful experience, even as I felt her frustration with her department. I suspected her co-workers were dismissive of her new hands-on approach to patients (physical therapy also was involved in the newer facilitation methods) and of her interest in group treatment. Marcia eventually resigned, and I continued the group sessions alone.

THE HARSH REALITIES OF THE ERA

My position at the state hospital ended unceremoniously. There is an ebb and flow in the life of all organisms and even in political and health systems. I did not know then that it was an ominous preview of what would occur two decades later with downsizing and mergers. After all, this was a setting where everyone felt very secure. Life in this hospital ebbed away.

My requests to attend workshops were first taken to the administrative assistant before the medical chief received them. One day when I went to register for funds and permission to attend a course, the administrative assistant stated with some hostility that I was always requesting money for a workshop and that others should have this opportunity. I agreed and asked whether others had done so. Was I taking more than my share and causing others to be turned away? She replied that even though few other requests had been made, and despite the availability of funds, it seemed unfair that I should benefit so often.

I was baffled, but I intended to persist. The opportunity never materialized. Both of us came to work the next day to learn that she, I, and everyone else in the hospital—doctors, nurses, clerical staff, professional staff—had lost our jobs! The state had decided to close down one of its hospitals, and ours was selected without any warning. It was a noiseless eruption. It felt like a death. We were the dead and the mourners, and there was no one to explain or give comfort. It was my first brush with an unfair, incomprehensible system where no one would ever provide an explanation. It was abandonment by a system that I had come to trust.

Everyone experienced shock and a deep sense of loss. We disbanded in 1975. I became too busy working on the problem and did not anticipate the dips and heights that any career journey takes. It need not seem like such a calamity. But my sensibilities were not developed to the degree required.

Confronting Sexism

It is well known how women in this era usually found insensitivity in the workplace, and it was difficult to negotiate for time off when it was necessary to be absent from work. An unrelenting tension always existed between my supervisors and me throughout this decade. And where could one talk about it, especially when there would be little empathy extended because of the prevailing attitude that mothers belonged at home? Society constantly expressed ambivalence for the working mother. As the mother of children who were then 8, 14, and 18 years old, I was keenly aware of a hostile climate for working mothers. This was not a time when juggling sicknesses, school events, or any other family matter was appreciated as natural to the daily life of working professionals. That is why I look with wonder and appreciation at the achievement of the Family and Medical Leave Act of 1993, which protects everyone who must maintain the tenuous balance of responding to family needs and working at a job.

As I looked for a reassignment in this kind of social climate, I saw that my choices were limited. I wanted to stay close to home, work in a hospital, and stay in the state system. This was what I knew. My family was my priority. Two of my children required hospitalizations for their escalating difficulty with Crohn's disease, and my parents were in their 90s, growing frail and needing more of my attention.

It was hardly a time for exploring professional options. I hung on to what I could of my sense of pleasure and interest in work by reading and talking with colleagues. I was aware that the predictable responsibilities I met at work, contrary to expectation, gave me an inner strength and confidence that carried over to decrease my sense of frustration in meeting the unpredictable needs of my family. My work offered satisfaction, although it might in fact have been a good time for a vacation.

It would have been nice to see the Little Mermaid sculpture in Denmark, or to pick flowers in the mountains in southern France, or to visit the Cloisters in nearby New York. But those seemed like indulgences. It was my habit to be practical, and I wanted to attend to responsibilities. The notion did occur to me, however, that the practical decision is not always the healthiest.

A New Hospital, a Renewed Purpose

Four months after my departure from Cedarcrest, I was offered a staff therapist's position at Connecticut Valley Hospital. The hospital had an excellent rehabilitation department that was administered by highly competent occupational therapists. The department had its own headquarters building and dedicated clinical areas in all the other buildings on the hospital grounds. The printing department was in the occupational therapy headquarters. I had visited in earlier decades, and I was delighted by the graphic arts area; it was my favorite craft.

The printing department was immense and well-equipped. Patients assigned for treatment produced all the hospital's print materials, including an impressive weekly newsletter. My first opportunity to be published occurred there.

I was aware that some civil rights groups considered as abusive the use of patient labor in the print shop, on the hospital's farm, and elsewhere in the facility. In later years, it would become another kind of conflicted situation. When laws prohibited the use of patients as workers, the outcome seemed to result in slovenliness in patients' appearance and behaviors. Boredom and a lack of routine could be observed, and that indicated another set of abuses. Programs to substitute for the loss of useful, even skilled, work had not been created to fill the gap of too much unstructured time for the hospital patient.

I was grateful for my new position and started again to be involved in full-time clinical treatment in an old building devoted to long-term care.

My space was in the basement—grim, dark, and damp. The walls and floors were discolored from time and from urine stains. Yet there was an element of grandeur in the high ceilings, the large windows, and the paneled walls of the main rooms.

The patients were mostly elderly, and the women and men were in separate wards. Most had been there for decades and probably would have felt uneasy in another setting. I noted that several had foot drop, an iatrogenic condition that occurs in patients who are strapped or restrained in chairs that are too high for the patient's feet to touch the floor. Over time, the ankle flexors stretch too much to recover, and standing upright and walking become impossible. Those patients had to crawl from place to place or always be in a wheelchair.

The facility's treatment style was purely custodial, and the mood on a ward depended on the congeniality or indifference of the nursing staff. Pathos and humor coexisted. I saw one elderly man pull at the locked door, "It's time for me to go home." "Of course," said the nurse supervisor pleasantly, "But we want you to stay for dinner, and you can think about leaving then." The place held fertile soil for an occupational therapist.

I decided to continue where I had left off at Cedarcrest, and I began working with patients on ADLs: bathing, dressing, and grooming. In the mornings, I went to the lavatories to help the nurses, who performed those activities with large groups of patients. The nurses appreciated the assistance, although our approaches were different. I would persuade and guide a few patients to do their own care, while the nurses performed total care on a large number.

The patients at Cedarcrest had physical traumas or diseases that resulted in a range of losses. A brain injury could damage the ability to remember the sequence of bathing or dressing. Some physical loss—of a limb, perhaps—or dysfunction that caused limited movement, or other impairment like severe arthritis would require either retraining in another method to accomplish ADLs or learning to use adaptive equipment. At the Connecticut Valley Hospital, there were patients with the same conditions, but for others the chief requirements were to rekindle motivation, to review the sequencing of procedures, and to support their efforts with practice.

The morning readiness program was bedlam. Many personalities, with their moods and idiosyncrasies, were crowded into a tiled, noisy space. The odors were noxious, and there was a general shortage of supplies that required creative substitutions. There was no one to hand out towels, washcloths, or underwear. Personality clashes occurred all the time. But miracles also occurred. At the end of a relatively short period, from the confusion there emerged our patients, clean, dressed, and groomed—shining wonders to behold. I felt accomplished. I felt welcomed. I felt a part of One Grand Production. I heard a drum roll!

As I worked with the nurses each morning, I did not know that I would reap a tremendous advantage, and disadvantage, as a consequence. My peers in the occupational therapy department did not share my interest in this activity. Working in the bathrooms on ADLs had never been a part of the program, although I did not know that. My colleagues avoided me, and I speculated that my morning work and some of my other beliefs contributed to their behavior.

It was not an environment where I would feel safe to speak openly as I had been in my first position at the Board of Education and Services for the Blind. However, there were many other positives in this situation to content me. A decade or so later, a new occupational therapy staff, all of them graduating with modern credentials, would institute an ADL program.

Becoming a Partner in Group Therapy

I continued working on my concept of group therapy. Every patient looked old, but not all of them were. They had aged as a result of stress imposed by many years of illness and the debilitating effect of long-term use of psychotropic drugs. Most were chronic patients, following the regulations passively, spending time staring into space, pacing, perhaps talking to themselves, sometimes screaming. When patients became disruptive, they would either be removed from the day room or be placed in a "geri-chair," a high-backed armchair that had a sliding tray in front to keep the patient locked in a sitting position. Some people were tied into their wheelchairs with cloth posies. The *posey* was a cloth device that fit over the chest and front upper torso restraining the arms and tied tightly in the back around neck and back to prevent a person from exiting the wheelchair. It was possible for a small, thin, or overactive adult to struggle and get caught in the wrapping and be choked to death or lose consciousness. These posies eventually were outlawed. Perhaps 15 to 20 patients were in the room when I would start my group.

I created a circle with the four or five who seemed most alert. I made a larger circle of the remaining folk and placed them behind us and around us to watch, to sleep, or even to interact when possible. To each member of the inner circle I held out my hand, and smiling, tried to make eye contact. I had the sensation of watching a flock of ducks swimming away in another direction at my approach to feed them!

I did not feel adequate, but I strenuously tried to override this feeling and to persist with the group. I brought pictures to show and crafts people could work with easily on their chair trays. I introduced an exercise for them to follow or tried to ask questions that would lead to conversation. It was important to me to get to know them as individuals, and that was difficult because they were not interested in me and had long since abandoned, in spirit at least, their external environment.

Their desolation challenged my ideas of the good life. I wanted to understand why they had given up, and I looked at them not as shadows but as real people from whom to ask sensible questions. My curiosity stirred up what Csikszentmihalyi (1993) later called a sense of *flow*, an absorption in what I was doing.

Bringing any item required watchfulness; some patients might try to eat it. Reaching to shake hands was risky, too; some might hit or grab my hand to twist my fingers. I soon learned to extend only my index and middle fingers as this made it easier for me to withdraw if someone attempted to tighten his or her grasp. Spitting or kicking, while not necessarily vindictive, could be forthcoming, and I watched for this possibility. At first, I often was ignored. In general, the group was not accustomed to attention, and most of them had long forgotten that personal attention is rewarding.

Nevertheless, as the months passed I learned which patients could respond and what item, activity, or sensation might cause them to respond. The nurses encouraged me. I particularly liked the head nurse for her wit and respectful handling of the patients. In general, the nursing staff was glad that the patients were getting attention. Many of them demonstrated a caring and protective quality in their service. Fortunately for me, they did not criticize what I was doing but praised me for getting any reaction.

Ruby, a group member in her 60s, was one patient with whom I could interact in instruction on self-care. She was feisty, she pretended senility and incompetence, and she enjoyed feigning helplessness. Still, she was quite strong and made interesting observations. During one group session we were reading a short poem extolling freedom and the ability to fly in space, going where our fancies took us. If they could leave, the group members assured me—and Ruby did so in particular—they would do so only to return to the hospital, their home of choice at the end of the day.

Another time as I was working alone with Ruby, I complimented her on her progress in bathing and dressing herself. She spoke sharply to me, "All my life I worked hard, and I am entitled to be waited on now." She saw the hospital as her reward, and she resented having to help herself. I am quite sure she retreated to that when I left her ward.

Patients, residents, clients—people in general—are shaped by culture. Place them in a totally custodial environment, and they lose all individuality or desire for meaningful activity. Thus it is that—although I had contact with many—there are few individual stories about patients who would allow intimacy or closeness in contact or who were able to continue with an activity on their own. I still felt encouraged by the slightest gain.

Although I did not know it then, my persistence was on the right track. Just 5 years later, there would be a great effort made to move patients like mine from hospitals to nursing homes in the community (Padilla, 2005c). The new belief was that being in the community would offer an environment that allowed more freedom and stimulation. Formal programs similar to mine were created and implemented to help patients make the change, eventually resulting in far lower patient populations in psychiatric hospitals.

At the same time, I began to seek group experiences for myself outside of work. I found to my consternation that I was generally uneasy in a group. I began to think, "What am I doing conducting groups, creating my ideas about their formation, while I am resisting groups myself?" When I joined a group, I would block my feelings. I felt inhibited, but mostly I wondered what was expected of me. I had thought being in a group was so natural it would be easy. Instead, I was worried about how I acted or what others might think. I knew that personal growth often comes from discomfort, so I persisted. I soon learned that I was very much like the rest of the human race, thinking I was inadequate or afraid I would say the wrong thing and believing all the while that others had more to offer. I gradually overcame my self-consciousness as my discomfort made me realize that others coming to my groups also were bringing their individual reactions and must find awareness and empathy in me.

The books, courses, and programs that are so prevalent now were not readily available in the mid-1970s. However, the groups I could find helped me to recognize my feelings and to examine the role I wanted to assume in the groups I conducted. My ideas changed over the years as I joined different groups: gestalt, bioenergetics, encounter, recovery, and spirituality (Lowen, 1966; Smith, 1976; Yalom, 1983). In conducting group sessions, I first saw myself as a helper or partner, then as a facilitator and, in moments of euphoria, even as a healer. Sometimes, it felt as though I were "sculpting" a group, creating desirable outcomes with calming or alerting techniques. Considering the leader as a coach also is very applicable in working with such groups. "Partner" is probably the way I saw myself most often in the clinical setting.

Because they were activity based, my groups were not designed for psychotherapy. Rather, I was a partner willing to work with others to explore, to consider, and to share in working out the problems that arose during the time of meeting. One cannot escape learning more about oneself as a member or as a leader of a group.

Collaborating With a New Mentor and Kindred Spirits

About a year after my arrival, the department got a new director, Brenda Smaga, OTR, MS. Brenda had organizational brilliance and took the reins with high velocity. She could keep three secretaries busy and presided over a challenging staff of 55. She also was a very active member of the ConnOTA, receiving throughout the ensuing years many awards of appreciation. About two decades later, AOTA would honor her as a Fellow.

Brenda and I met in the basement of the hospital building where I worked, and I described my program to her. After visiting me, she started to walk back through the dark corridor. It must have struck her as a desolate and forbidding place. She stopped suddenly, and she seemed engulfed in the light of her energy and enthusiasm. She turned around and called loudly to me, "I know what you are doing here, Mildred; you are hiding! I need you to help me. I won't do it all alone." She had many ideas to implement, and she needed support and help. It was the beginning of a robust friendship and the acquisition of a choice mentor for me.

By 1977, my schedule changed as Brenda found plenty of fascinating assignments for me. The staff needed continuing education, and I contributed to the creation or revision of many policy manuals. I helped train or supervise staff and students. I also continued to explore and develop a method for a group structure that would be successful with patients who were difficult to engage. This can be discouraging to therapists, and some of our staff members canceled their patient groups as often as they could. By the end of the decade, I became more effective in conducting groups and sharing methods with others.

I enjoyed coordinating the hospital's resources and arranging large-scale programs. One particularly large event had 1,500 registrants participate in a full-day workshop on mental health issues. Excellent people from many departments in the hospital contributed their efforts.

Brenda had very good ideas. Although she had a tendency to move fast and with determination and confidence that gave a strong incentive to every demand, I soon came to understand that her approach really was partnership. She paid attention to the suggestions of others and brought out the best in everyone.

Once, after an in-service session I had provided to staff, I lamented to her that the reception had been very cool and, in my opinion, my efforts a failure. Her answer was, "How do you know, Mildred? How can anyone tell until 6 months down the line? Sometimes there is great enthusiasm, and 6 months later no one remembers what it was all about. Sometimes there is no enthusiasm, and 6 months later you find the ideas being used in practice." I have reflected on this remark many times.

Brenda invited outstanding occupational therapists to her department. One such visitor was Lela A. Llorens, OTR, PhD, FAOTA, who had in 1969 delivered the Eleanor Clarke Slagle Lecture, occupational therapy's highest honor and recognition of scholarship. Her valuable theories and many publications have established a legacy in occupational therapy. On several occasions, such as when I was preparing for conferences, I found her very gracious to approach for counsel. She could be challenging but always understanding and encouraging. She has left an indelible impression on me as a rare person to admire. I met her half a dozen times to listen to her speak or to consult with her. She was gracious and wise but down to earth in her readiness to share herself. She understood well how intimacy and connection might be used to make sharing worthwhile.

One year we were planning an important statewide workshop at the hospital. A renowned occupational therapist, whom everyone wanted to host, had agreed to come. ConnOTA had informed Brenda that we should allow the association to host that dignitary rather than having her come to us. When I heard that, I became anxious; in my eagerness to bring this luminary to our hospital, I had completed almost all of the arrangements. I went to Brenda for a decision on the matter. With an impish look, she told me to continue with the arrangements. I admired her courage in light of the pressure put upon her. There were no repercussions; we had made a sensible decision.

It was at that well-attended workshop that much of my thinking about group conduct, theory, and methodology came together. The lectures were dynamic, combining neurology, physiology, learning theory, and approaches to activities that facilitate calm and alert behaviors or create chaos and anxiety. It helped clarify the swirling miasma of results I observed in my groups. The speaker, Lorna Jean King, was very knowledgeable—an inspired and inspiring occupational therapist exemplifying originality in thought and vivacity in delivery. I was fascinated.

Ms. King listed some principles for engaging patients with pervasive long-term mental illness. She described their slumped postures and apathetic behavior and the sudden change to more animated response that occurred when offered approaches based on her theories. Then she said that therapists should be eclectic and creative in compiling programs to help those patients change, and that we should draw from what we know about neurology and physiology. "But," she cautioned, "don't write a recipe book."

Never having thought about it before, I snapped to and said excitedly to myself, "Why not?" Why can't a carefully written recipe book encourage a free spirit in the clinic? Perhaps producing a fundamental structure that still had many options for therapists might be helpful. Allowing for flexibility within a structured framework is not necessarily a one-size-fits-all approach. Ms. King's cautionary advice was wise.

I made a short outline in a pamplet of a model I called the Five-Stage Group (Ross & Burdick, 1978). Each stage had a stated, intended purpose. How each stage was enacted depended on the therapist's particular interests and talents because so many tasks and activities can achieve similar goals. Each stage was equally important, and the cumulative effect of the stages would be the expected outcome of calm and alert behavior in group members.

Brenda began to assign other staff members to help with my groups. Often, staff people who did not want to plan the group were willing to participate once the group began. I wanted their observations, their intuitive reaction to the group session when it was over. It was a way for me to learn what I might not discern alone. Doris Kutyla, COTA, a very likable therapy assistant, worked with me for a time. One day after we completed our work with a group, I observed that the outcome was awful. Patients appeared confused and unresponsive. "What do you think was wrong?" I asked. "You pitched it too high, Mildred." I knew immediately that Doris's forthright statement was correct. That helped me to begin to strive very consciously for simplicity in task and presentation. I felt Mr. Ryan's presence and the memory of what he taught me about simplification and about getting the best result with the most economical effort.

I tried hard to emphasize that valuable quality in future workshops. Using slide presentations, I demonstrated how the simplest instructions brought a strong compliant response from group members. Usually that meant the activity was easily understood and had a bit of novelty that combined to make it irresistible.

Ellen Ashkins, a registered music therapist, worked with me on one of the toughest wards in the hospital. Violence and chaos existed on this ward of women, some of whom had been hospitalized for decades. Ellen was the exception to all the others who waited for me to plan and produce a group. Understanding my five-stage approach, she wanted to plan each group and discuss it with me afterward. She was a gifted musician and an outstanding therapist. I benefited greatly from our relationship and have the greatest admiration for music therapy. Several years later, when working at another facility with residents who had dementia, she would demonstrate the Five-Stage Group Model chiefly using music, and she contributed an excellent chapter to my 1987 book on group process (Ross, 1987).

Dona Burdick was a recreational therapist at the Connecticut Valley Hospital who also had a master's degree in physical education. For several years, she had treated the same population with whom I had chosen to work. I did not meet her right away; she was assigned to a different building on the hospital grounds. When we did meet, I found a kindred spirit. She was excited by the explanation of sensory integration principles, and we had a wonderful time sharing our interests. Her teaching expertise amazed me. She would help me get adults safely onto large therapeutic balls (in that era they were used chiefly with children), achieve their cooperation, and watch their pleasure at gently rocking on the balls for vestibular stimulation. Our patients enjoyed the activity, and it helped them to have more control of their behavior during group time.

Later, we ordered custom-made, adult-size scooter boards and other equipment with which we could experiment in our effort to decrease the chaotic behaviors in the group work we conducted together. Our collaborative work with the groups was always rewarding. Dona's expertise was in movement, and she could design the entire five stages in movement to express perception and reflection as well as closure. Her name is on the first manual and the first manuscript that I wrote (Ross & Burdick, 1981).

The collaborations with Ellen and Dona were important because the enthusiastic interchange of ideas and expertise helped all of us in our work. We found that, together, we could have a quieting and organizing effect on the patients.

Because students also were assigned to work with me, I found myself using the same information and the same encouraging cues to stimulate their creativity and share my concerns about what patients needed. I approached Brenda with a short manual I had been providing to students. I proposed that I could expand it and suggested that the hospital could print and sell it, using the profits to fund whatever was needed. It was my desire to share with anyone who wanted ideas about groups. At the time there were very few books that explained how to apply theory to practice. Brenda approved the project, and the print shop produced it. In 1978, about 3,000 manuals were sold throughout the country at $3 per copy; some copies are still floating around today (Ross & Burdick, 1978).

It is impossible to provide an exact recipe for every group because each time a group meets it can present the facilitator with a new configuration of needs, responses, and environmental variables. The five stages provide an outline for orientation, movement, perceptual tasks, reflection, and closure. The interests and skills of the therapists and the presenting needs of members fill in the content. The manual also had suggestions for content.

The same five-stage structure and principles are followed today. The tasks employed within the progressively demanding stages must and do change with the years to maintain relevance to and keep abreast of the interests of group participants.

I was immeasurably grateful to the hospital for its bountiful resources. The audiovisual director, Arnold Eastman, lent his tremendous skill in videotaping group sessions. He also photographed sessions to develop a slide presentation of the method. He was an expert photographer who caught spontaneous expressions, positions of hands, and nurturing gestures of group members to show the drama and emotion stimulated within each stage. His pictures and photographed illustrations for the manual and workshops resulted in a truly moving, first-rate product. It was a privilege to watch and to work with him during that part of his long and distinguished career in state service. He helped me organize workshops at the hospital and prepare slide presentations of many group sessions.

THE OCCUPATIONAL THERAPIST IN CHARGE

The late 1970s marked the beginning of the final hour for the season of occupational therapy's dominance in the rehabilitation world of mental health treatment. It had been an accepted understanding that a registered occupational therapist directed large departments and that occupational therapists were to receive supervision only from other occupational therapists. Beginning in the early 1980s, occupational therapy lost that distinction. A more egalitarian attitude made it possible for recreation, music, dance, horticulture, and vocational rehabilitation therapists to supervise the rehabilitation treatment in mental health. It is now commonplace for professionals in different therapeutic disciplines, including physical therapy, to supervise each other even though each profession approaches specific treatment differently.

Sharing and learning from one another is a good way to coordinate treatment, but supervision must suffer. In my opinion, each professional practice is unique and grows chiefly from a dialogue emerging from its own roots. It benefits from supervision provided by a member of that profession.

The repercussions from the new approach did not show immediately. For another decade and a half, during the 1980s and the first half of the 1990s, occupational therapists would remain in demand, and salaries swelled as good job opportunities were available.

Getting an Opportunity to Contribute to Change

Connecticut Valley Hospital offered daily adventures, but there were vexations, too. The administrative groups in the various buildings were constantly in flux and, as is typical of a bureaucracy, that threatened the stability of any agenda. A program or a building might be closed without warning. A promotion might take an ideal supervisor away from a program, killing a schedule that was working. However, sometimes a new person enters who contributes to a fresh start.

Such a situation was the arrival of a physician, Benjamin MacDonald, MD, who eventually visited the building where I worked with my groups. We had stimulating conversations about the hospital, the patients, and his ideas for providing medical care. He had accepted the post of unit chief of the psychogeriatric program in the newly renovated Woodward Hall, and in an unprecedented move, he asked that I be appointed as his assistant unit chief. This was in 1977 and 1978. In the history of the hospital, only a few women had ever held that title, and certainly no one did who was not a physician. The medical director, who also was the superintendent, approved my appointment. It was my opportunity to contribute to changes I had always wanted to see become a reality for the geriatric population.

I was pleased and flattered. I hardly noticed that no one mentioned any increase in my salary. Brenda retained some of my time but finally replaced me with a new young therapist, Valnere McLean, OTR, whom I began to know as a valuable ally. She was a good friend in the rehabilitation department, and throughout the years I would greatly benefit from her foresight and resourcefulness. In the years to follow she achieved an MS, a BCN (board certification in neurology), and also an FAOTA.

Valnere acquired compassion, flexibility, and tolerance in her views from her background. She was born in India to American parents and educated in Australia. She lived on at least four continents during her marriage. Valnere contributed greatly to occupational therapy services in the hospital. Graduating in 1975 with a degree in occupational therapy, she joined ConnOTA, working ardently for the next 15 years for its successes and receiving many awards. Valnere is part of the history of ConnOTA as she was co-chair of the Government Affairs Committee and, once licensure passed in 1979, was one of the people instrumental in achieving reimbursement for occupational therapists. As the alternate in the Representative Assembly with Virginia Rollefson, OTR/L, MS, she remained very involved, and in her post in government affairs, with Irene Herden, OTR/L, MBA, FAOTA, she achieved the hiring of a lobbyist in the 1980s that has been an exceptional benefit to ConnOTA to this day. Irene, too, has worked tirelessly for decades for ConnOTA and is still doing so.

Even as I threw myself into the many administrative details of the new Woodward Hall, I continued to conduct groups in other buildings. One day, Woodward Hall's therapist generously allowed Mr. Eastman to tape a group that we were conducting together. Practicing the Five-Stage Group Model whenever possible had become a habit for me. It helped me get to know the patients as people. On this day, a near-disaster occurred right at the beginning. As I directed simple movement and all the members complied, one woman turned on me with resentment. I had mistakenly touched her on the shoulder without first asking permission. Lucy rose from her chair and, with rising anger, shook her finger in my face. I thought she might strike me. My expression (shown in the film) was full of regret at what I had done. When she finished her complaint, I asked her what she wanted to do, whether to stay or leave. She left. To regroup, I did not trivialize the incident; I assured everyone that Lucy would be missed but that I had learned something that I would never repeat. I began another activity that I hoped would interest everyone, and it did; the group carried on successfully. There was a longer term benefit from the experience: I used the slides from that session in one of my books.

When the session ended, I went to the ward to find Lucy. I asked her what had made her so angry. She stated that I had requested group members after shaking a neighbor's hand to reach forward and tap one shoulder. However, her partner would not do this. It was at that moment that I had touched her, but she had wanted her partner—a man—to do this! She had a natural, innocent desire to participate in the activity. I explained that her partner was too cognitively impaired to understand the request. My guess was that, had he understood, he would have liked to participate effectively. Lucy had considered it a rejection, not realizing that when I at first requested partners shake hands, she had started the movement for him so that he did not seem so impaired. I explained that he had to initiate the second part of the activity but did not understand how to do that. A few days later, Lucy was discharged, apparently because she seemed much more responsive than she had been. It was almost as though she had been awakened by the episode and had become able to make decisions. I believe it was helpful for Lucy to express herself and to show her feelings; she had been unaccustomed to doing so. Again, I saw the value of people coming together to meet, act, and react to a group format.

Implementing the Personalized Care Model

The proverbial chickens came home to roost. The head nurse in Woodward Hall, Dolores Boccacio, RN, was the same head nurse with whom I had worked previously, so it was easier for me to be accepted by the newly assigned nursing staff, whose cooperation I needed. She told the nurses that I had taken my turn working with patients right alongside with the staff in the lavatories. I was appreciated for this.

The unit chief, the head nurse, and Helen Deag, the administrative assistant whose trusted advice I needed often, were all outstanding individuals who kept the business of Woodward moving forward. That progress was noticed. Less than a year later, Dr. MacDonald was promoted as assistant to the medical director in the main administrative building.

Before Dr. MacDonald left, he persuaded his colleague, Francisco Quintana, MD, to take his place. I had four more years of a good working relationship as assistant unit chief. Shortly after Dr. Quintana's arrival, a new program, the personalized care model (PCM) was proposed for all of the state's psychiatric hospitals. The PCM was an assessment and a plan for changes in hospital care to facilitate discharge to the community. It was a bold new idea that had developed outside the medical discipline. A New York anthropologist had introduced it as a way to facilitate the discharge of patients and to stop the revolving door of discharge and readmission of patients (Nicholson, 1968, 1975; Nicholson & Nicholson, 1982).

As the prevailing belief—that mental illness meant lifetime incarceration—changed, largely because of the availability of more effective drugs, more patients were discharged and changes in the community had to happen. However, the communities that received discharged patients had not developed sufficient and suitable programs for those people. It was now perceived that the hospital could help the community learn how to welcome those new residents as well as to prepare the patients in new and different ways for discharge.

Historically, it is interesting to review any great societal change to see how the many parts must be organized separately at first for each factor to merge into the whole. After separate progress, each part then must be coordinated for integration. Thorough cooperation is required to help the needed change become the new reality. In this instance, community organizations had to learn how to work with hospitals. And the hospitals had to change and work with patients differently to assist their readiness for the community.

The PCM was a systems change that instigated a total restructuring of mental health care. It changed the relationship of the staff in their interactions with one another and with patients. It required a total revamping of every aspect of patient treatment by all staff, especially psychiatric aides, whose duties expanded markedly. The model fulfilled all the requirements considered necessary for changing an inadequate program to respond to a broader societal need. It encompassed intensive education, environmental change, and constant reassessment of progress. To facilitate staff education, my duties included hosting professional trainers, creating a physical environment that provided stimulation and safety, and collaborating with those in other disciplines to tailor patient-specific treatment. My training in occupational therapy was a great benefit.

The primary care staff members needed to learn how to be therapeutically interactive with each patient. Although many of them had demonstrated a strong desire to work that way, they had not been encouraged or trained to do so. Consistent committee meetings would be required to keep all of this in place. The State Department of Mental Health mandated the program for our new geriatric facility and for the geriatric unit of another large state psychiatric facility. Today, many of the PCM constructs are taken for granted, but it was a new approach for everyone in the late 1970s.

The task was formidable and would require preparation on my part. Although I believed in the model, I had little faith that the implementation I was expected to conduct would receive the extensive long-term support it required. I requested an interview with the hospital's medical director to discuss the PCM plan.

I briefly reviewed the plan and confessed that I had little faith in the larger system, which frequently started new programs only to drop them when any other plan came along. I asked him for reassurance of his commitment to the program. Intensive work was required for results, and that would require support from the top down. He assured me that he was solidly behind the program, and I believed him. He remained true to his word, but future events would trump his decision.

PCM implementation in the geriatric facility was a bracing, exciting, and interesting time for everyone. As more doctors recognized and published on the subject of geriatrics in the late 1960s and 1970s, the conviction had grown that geriatric patients required special attention in practice. It is only in the past 25 years that geriatric medicine has gained a strong, accepted foothold. For example, it took until 1991 for the American Board of Psychiatry and Neurology (n.d.) to designate geriatric psychiatry as a separate specialty. At the time of this inquiry, I was told that, to be recognized as a geriatric psychiatrist, one must spend 4 years in medical school, 4 years in a postgraduate residency in psychiatry, 1 or 2 years in an intensive fellowship in geriatric psychiatry, and then pass certification examinations in general and in geriatric psychiatry.

In the 1970s, Connecticut Valley Hospital had an education program in mental health for medical residents. The psychiatrist in charge of the program asked me for suggestions and speakers that would stimulate interest in geriatrics. I could recommend physicians and other professionals available at the time to present information about sensory changes and sensory deprivation, perceptual disturbances, and physiological changes in the elderly population and how those factors influenced behavior. Whenever possible, I would talk with the medical residents about occupational therapy, as would other therapists. Not all hospitals in this era helped residents understand how to use occupational therapy.

The environment hummed. All staff, from maintenance to professional personnel, required some amount of re-education as new and expanded job roles were visualized for everyone. The nursing staff, at the center of this plan, began to understand that their attitude and behavior had to change to elicit new behaviors from patients. They also needed to acquire additional skills. It was my duty to arrange for that new learning in classes either scheduled in our building or at the state university, where a state grant was funding more courses on the PCM program.

Today, we assume that everyone in contact with patients should have strong interpersonal skills, but in the late 1970s, that principle of the PCM had to be instilled. The adoption of the model expanded the role of nursing assistants by making psychiatric aides the primary caregivers while increasing their accountability and control over the work setting. All of those lines of authority and responsibility were new.

Once the planning stage of assessment, goal establishment, and staff development sessions was completed, implementation began by assigning specific patients to specific staff who would be responsible for them. Nurses and aides were involved in a treatment schedule consisting of group treatment sessions that they could provide and identify as beneficial to patients. Setting the schedule and training the aides to conduct group sessions with which they felt comfortable were exciting for me. A background in occupational therapy is very suitable for these tasks. The aides decided to provide exercise, arts and crafts, games, grooming skills training, parties, timely discussions, and daily news sharing. The aides were very interested in the methods for planning and implementing this whole new set of skills they were acquiring. For several years, the daily calendar of events provided by a supportive nursing staff on each ward in Woodward Hall was the envy of staff members in the rest of the hospital.

I see the PCM, a systems change, as having broad implications for any kind of planned change, personal or external. Its strategy is to assess needs and decide on goals; create plans to meet the goals; and implement, reassess, and make adaptive changes continuously to those goals—all while keeping in touch with everyone involved. This is very similar to a treatment plan for occupational therapy. In our discipline, the therapist must be astutely aware of the vast range of ways to assess and meet individual needs.

As assistant unit chief, I could obtain equipment and supplies that were required for treatment by nursing staff. I requisitioned the maintenance staff to build a set of parallel bars (then considered essential) for treating patients recovering from strokes or amputations. When the nursing staff suggested we have our own gated area for outdoor picnics, I requested one to be constructed. Morale was greatly boosted when staff members could see the patients in their care enjoying themselves safely outside. I did research to determine whether linoleum or rugs would provide the better surface in our foyer. The nursing staff suggested that noxious odors should be ameliorated, and we worked with maintenance to resolve the problem.

The process of change can and did create frustration. The change that was expected was massive for a setting that had provided custodial care. Not everyone found the new requirements of the program acceptable. Some staff members departed; a few tried to sabotage the program. This was true of therapists also and was met by daily restatements about what was expected. There is no other recourse in state service because it is almost impossible for anyone to be fired. In general, everyone grew more competent as they contributed to the success of the program, and they were acknowledged for this. It was a stimulating process.

Nursing homes have different selection criteria, so the working strategy is to focus on what the patient needs to acquire to be discharged. That is accomplished by creating a triangle of physician, nurse, and nursing assistant to act as a liaison between community and hospital, and nurses become experts on the different styles of the local facilities. The local nursing homes are briefed about the patient ready for discharge. They are assured that the unit chief, the psychiatrist, is quick to respond to questions and to warn the nursing home of symptoms new patients might have. A close alliance is worked out with the community, and problems are headed off by swift consultation between the community residence and the hospital. In this way, preventive care is used more often than crisis management to produce successful outcomes. The unit chief is on call for the nursing home not only to help sustain the placement but to be ready to say when the patient should be returned. Everyone works to benefit the whole program, including the patient, who is helped to see choices that exist.

I saw sick men and women getting better and recovering enough to be discharged willingly. The rate of readmission in geriatrics plummeted!

chapter 5

THE 1980S:
DEVELOPMENTAL DISABILITIES

CONSEQUENCES OF COST-CUTTING

Honored While Losing Ground

In the midst of our energetic endeavors, stunning news arrived at Woodward Hall in 1981. State officials had dismissed the medical director who had headed the hospital for several decades. As far as I knew, he had been responding with integrity and openness to patients and staff. Although I always felt the inner workings of the hospital pulse through me, I did not have a clue about the political reasons for his dismissal. I was very sorry and immediately understood that our program had lost its assurance of security.

At the same time, the hospital authorities set in motion a huge celebration for all hospital staff that seemed a bewildering contrast to the existing grave uncertainties. Were they the Romans, giving us circuses for distraction? Or were they providing the condemned with a favorite last meal?

As we assembled at banquet tables in a huge dining hall, we were to witness the honoring of 11 employees selected from almost 1,100 hospital personnel. Sitting at an assigned table, I looked around and realized how much I appreciated the people I recognized from other departments. They had given me so much help and support during the 7 years before. It was a heartwarming, down-to-earth event. Among the first honorees was a gentle, modest man from the maintenance department, who was recognized as outstanding for his enduring dependability.

Each department, I learned, had chosen one person to be honored. Unknown to me, Brenda Smaga had offered my name. When toward the end I was called up, I was completely surprised. As I walked toward the master of ceremonies and turned, I saw the psychology department staff rise to their feet and applaud. This distinctive action, provided no one else, made an indelible impression on me. I felt immensely warmed, as there had been a lot of good interaction over the years. That wonderful moment, that surge of good feeling, is a lasting memory. I returned to my table holding the commemorative plaque. The oddity of the occasion did not manifest itself until a short time later.

The new superintendent lost no time in identifying a list of important issues to pursue, but neither our building nor our geriatric service was assessed for progress or contributions. Rather, Dr. Quintana was called to task for working with an assistant who was neither male nor a physician. Because Dr. Quintana would not replace me, he was given the option of transferring to another building. He refused. Dr. Quintana voiced the unfairness of our situation to me. However, I could not help but observe some disconnect from our previous close relationship. Even as I tried to deny it, I was becoming vulnerable to the attack set in motion by the new superintendent.

The superintendent had his way. A few months later, Dr. Quintana chose to leave the hospital, taking a position in a state hospital in another town, and I was required to return full time as a staff therapist in the Rehabilitation Department. The Woodward Hall program had had two invested psychiatrists for 5 years. At least nine psychiatrists came and went during the next 2 years. To my knowledge, no assistant unit chief was appointed again.

The day of successful court cases on gender bias and even age bias was still to dawn. It was 1982, and I lacked the vigor and the historical precedent to struggle against this kind of injustice. However, I recognized then that I had had enough of state service.

My friends at the hospital supported me in every way they could, yet I felt as abandoned and isolated as I did during the earlier hospital closing in 1975. Shortly after returning to the Rehabilitation Department, I met an occupational therapist who, seeing me, said, probably humorously but pointedly, "Well, Mildred, you're nobody now!" A psychologist I had counted as a friend called me to ask how it felt to have "lost face." Neither comment adequately reflected my feelings; the elation of the administrative opportunity afforded me would never leave me, even as I felt my present disappointment.

The remarks reminded me of a scene in the 1962 movie of the Harper Lee (1960) novel *To Kill a Mockingbird* (Pakula & Mulligan). Tom Robinson, a black man falsely accused of raping a white woman, is defended by Atticus Finch, a well-respected white lawyer who loses the case, despite his eloquence and command of the facts. Others asked the Finch children, "Didn't it make us mad to see our daddy beat?" That question somehow shifts the focus of the failure from those who perpetuate an immoral system—and the failure of that system to be fair—to one man as he stands up to the system alone. I believed I had been wronged because of a lack of ethics in the system, and I felt no blame for not being able to continue my role.

I missed the work I so much enjoyed, and I worried that the benefits to the patients of our building's achievements might drain away. I felt thrown off base, and I knew how quickly the rushing waters of the next event would roll over us so that everything would be soon forgotten.

Leaving State Service

I returned to documenting those groups I was still permitted to lead in the occupational therapy department. I also was assigned to accompany large groups of patients on outings, an activity for which I was not very suited and did not like. Still, it was familiar work and, as my father always said, "All work is honorable." But I was working with a numbed spirit, and I lacked a sense of flow. It became possible to think of moving away to another setting. I was learning about bringing more detachment to my work. I was seeing each generation of changing leaders in a bureaucracy bring an even more stark inadequacy to the charge to serve. Appointees at the top made decisions with little knowledge, seeking little information in support of the common good beyond the balance sheets that show the fastest way to cut costs.

Now every department in the hospital reflected a need to run for cover in response to the hatchet the new superintendent wielded. As everyone began to feel unsafe, there was less lively sharing among departments. The psychiatrist whose charge was to create programs for continuing education for residents found his hours cut and his decision making severely restricted. The new superintendent put in different standards and priorities for all staff. He imposed them in a cunning manner. From the very beginning when I had gone to him, he had acted as if he could not understand my uneasiness. He would reassure me that he had heard good things about my work and that he was not contemplating changes. He continually lied to me with a direct and kindly expression, as he did with others.

The hospital's patients suffer the most when there is a turnabout in policies. Unexpected changes and unpredictable events cause anxiety among staff members. And staff members are less patient and use fewer preventive measures when interacting with and calming patients. Patients perceive change they cannot understand because there are never any explanations. Patients and staff members feel destabilized and confused and search for equilibrium with a variety of coping measures that drain their energy. All of this is part of a predictable cycle in state institutions.

Not only does the pattern of chaos occur in state institutions, it happens in agencies and in corporations that lack systems of checks and balances. Ironically, it sometimes appears to be the very way society must struggle to make progress! As the wrong and destructive way of doing business becomes intolerable, it allows collaborative, cooperative, creative forces to have a chance to lead with improved approaches. This was after all how PCM had come into being. But over time, some small corruption begins even in the new and improved design, and the cycle continues. Apathy and cynicism take root, and workers can lose patience for the big picture or the long wait. No matter what the positive results over the long haul, it is a creeping and grim way to achieve progress.

For me it was a recollection of my time at the Board of Education and Services for the Blind when Mr. Ryan was replaced by a self-seeking, smooth-talking, indifferent director, who eventually proved incompetent. In like manner, the new superintendent at Connecticut Valley Hospital would serve 5 years before he, too, would be removed under a cloud. When one can look back, it can be seen that justice does triumph—just enough to make sense. But usually it's too late for those who are sacrificed.

Brenda Smaga moved on to another opportunity. A rehabilitation supervisor—a recreational therapist—was appointed by the new superintendent to lead the department. The new age of putting everything under activity therapy, of mix-and-match supervisors for manifold therapies, had arrived. The new supervisor was intelligent but not very interested in her work. The quality of the department's work fell. I secured a small state retirement package that did not reflect the 30 years I had worked in state hospitals. I had taken many summers and some years off to be with my children, and I was penalized for not being at retirement age. Within the year, I departed to try private practice and looked forward to the opportunity to be almost exclusively with my clients. I soon learned that the community provided infinite possibilities; I wondered why I had waited so long.

The passing of time brought some gleeful events. In 2001 I was invited—and paid well—to present a day-and-a-half workshop at Connecticut Valley Hospital on the Five-Stage Group Model. Therapists, nurses, and physicians attended. In 2004, a friend informed me that a special room with sensory modalities in the Learning Center of the hospital had been named after me.

PRIVATE PRACTICE AND THE COMMUNITY

As emerging concepts opened new doors, the community was ready to offer many possibilities to the individual therapist seeking private practice. Health care costs had continued to rise in the 1980s, which influenced a shift toward cost containment for hospitals and shorter hospital stays (Struthers & Boyt Schell, 1991). Mechanisms were put in place to provide payment for specialized services such as occupational therapy treatment, including funding for educating children who were handicapped, in which occupational therapy was covered as a related service (Education for All Handicapped Children Act of 1975; Amendments to the Education of the Handicapped Act, 1986), and coverage for occupational therapy in outpatient settings, skilled nursing facilities, and private practice clinics (Struthers & Boyt Schell, 1991). The number of private practices greatly increased in the late 1980s and early 1990s, spurred by legislation that allowed occupational therapists to bill third party payers, such as Medicare and Medicaid (Bailey, 1998).

New occupational therapy graduates could choose supervisory positions in schools, in long-term care, and in home care that offered good pay and benefits (AOTA, 1985a). New kinds of residential living arrangements and more for-profit, long-term-care facilities were developed to house those released from institutions. Public education mainstreamed children with disabilities into the schools, although that did not mean that they learned alongside their peers; they were placed in separate rooms and took separate paths during the school day (Armstrong, 1996; Kavale, 2002).

Ordinarily, I would not have chosen to work in a regular school setting because I lacked adequate experience, but once children with severe disabilities were placed in the schools, I found that I had a store of useful, generic knowledge. My private practice had led to a contract with children with severe disabilities, so I was aware of their conditions as I concentrated on working with teachers and aides. Those teachers held my greatest admiration because of their genuine dedication to students who seemed to have no end of perplexing difficulties. I was well acquainted with the ideas of positioning, the teaching of self-soothing methods for self-abusing children, and the ways to use the results of sensory testing. I could add clarity to these areas.

As patients moved out of hospitals after shorter stays, new subacute treatment facilities began to multiply. The number of agencies that managed home care mushroomed (Evanofski, 2003). Residential group homes were created for the populations discharged from the now-shuttered institutions. (Planners had to learn the hard way that discharged patients required an introduction to home-like living, or an expensive facility might be destroyed. At first, a few group homes were set up for people with mental retardation who had been discharged from Mansfield Training Center, an entrenched and old institution where they may have lived all their lives. The new group homes were designed to include expensive furniture, décor, and fixtures not familiar to the newly transferred occupants. When disagreements occurred among the residents, the interior of these early extravagant homes might be trashed by them, because they knew few ways to control anger and anxieties.)

The exodus from the hospitals and institutions to the community created a Mecca for novice and experienced therapists as federal and state governments continued to mandate high-quality health care and to underwrite much of its cost. As enrollments grew, programs for teaching occupational therapy expanded, and there was a burgeoning market for workshop presenters and lecturers (AOTA, 1991). I, too, was swept along in a community jungle of infinite possibilities, and I prospered, believing it could only get better.

Seeking Possibilities in Private Practice

Colleagues and mentors recharged my professional life and helped me to move forward. One of them, Valnere McLain, also had resigned from the hospital to start a private practice. When an agency providing home care in my town offered her work too far from her home, she suggested my name. I began a part-time arrangement while still employed by the state hospital. When I left state service, I retained my agency affiliation.

Communities held many new opportunities. I found private schools, sheltered workshops, and nursing homes that wanted the services of an occupational therapist. I realized that my continuous attendance at educational conferences during my state service had kept me up to date, viable, and able to contribute.

Private enterprise was possible. Valnere and I formed a partnership with Virginia Rollefson, OTR/L, an occupational therapist known for her activism and work with children, to convene local workshops. That enterprise worked well for several years, and it enlightened me about business. When I had arranged workshops under the auspices of an institution, cost was not so much an issue and there were many departments to help me. It was quite different when the total cost and all the services involved had to be secured by very few people operating privately.

Among the first colleagues to arrange an out-of-state invitation was Anne Scott, OTR/L, PhD, FAOTA, who made it possible for me to provide workshops in New York. She created the occupational therapy program at the Brooklyn Campus of Long Island University. Anne has shared her knowledge in a variety of articles, chapters, and books and touched the lives of many occupational therapists and clients with her wisdom and support. A dear friend, Sharon Gresk, who in the early 1980s was president of the Connecticut Association of Therapeutic Recreation Directors, promoted my negotiation of contracts to present many workshops for this group. After a career change, Sharon now enjoys success as a freelance graphic artist. Other professions, including those who work in nursing, with Alzheimer's patients, or with adults with other cognitive disabilities, requested seminars illustrating the flexibility of the Five-Stage Group Model to achieve their professional needs.

Learning New Perspectives in Work Services

A part-time position 2 days each week that began in 1984 in a sheltered workshop, which now would be called *work services*, became the financial core of my practice. I treated people with mental retardation, developmental disabilities, autism, and other behavioral health difficulties.

In working with those populations, I found that it was easy either to underestimate or to overestimate abilities; each person has so many subtleties and complexities. Standardized assessments are not generally available and treatment demanded every skill I had ever acquired. When I departed years later, I discovered that I was rewarded with new competence and confidence because I had been much challenged by that work. All of those groups are excellent populations for teaching a therapist how to stretch.

It is generally accepted that every experience and each case we treat teaches and changes us. The population with developmental disabilities is no different. They teach by example. They express their feelings with hugs, tears, moving closer, pointing, or finding an unexpected small phrase for despair or pleasure, anger, or hurt. In contrast to those who verbalize everything, their simplicity brings a greater poignancy, directness, and earnestness to a situation. I wanted to respond to this with clear and plain language of my own. Imagine if this could be the way we operate in politics and business? That experience helped me simplify my own thinking, get to the core of an issue, and be direct in description or action.

There was another, deeper effect that population had on me. When I had to interact with them, I was compelled to grapple with my irritation and impatience, which I had recognized as arrogance. I began to gain a greater perspective on how responses could be understood from another person's point of view. I recognized that there are truly many ways to interpret all the information that bombards us. Problems are magnified especially when information is received through sensory systems that are impaired with possible problems in vision, hearing, or myriad other sensory perception areas.

This helped me appreciate all people—including myself. It furthered the path of "becoming" and showed how the work of occupational therapy is enriching in practice as it is in study. The field is so comprehensive, and our openness to it prepares us for this greater understanding.

Learning From Clients

Disturbances in the sensory systems are a part of mental retardation (Ross & Bachner, 2004). Fortunately, the occupational therapist is trained to understand how sensory disturbance influences behavior. Sometimes it is possible to see the humor: A "defect" in someone turns out to be so ordinary that each of us has it. For example, Goodwill Industries in my town had a large room devoted to collecting and arranging donated clothing. Sometimes, the clothing was jammed together on hangers that were hard to separate. A young client named Sally was given the task of shooting a price tag into the sleeves of garments. The staff members reported that she could not locate the sleeve or the seam very often, although she could use the gun adequately. They had heard about perceptual problems and presented Sally to me for an assessment. My assessment was almost instant: She needed adequate light in her work area. As soon as that was improved, Sally's "visual and tactile perceptual problems" disappeared. Even if she had known she could ask for better light in the workroom, Sally was very likely too timid to do so. This episode once again made me realize how important it is to understand one's rights.

There are many examples of parents who provide a loving, caring home to children with developmental disabilities, but most of the clients I saw in work services had known only institutional care, where uniformity is expected and natural spontaneity is restricted. Most of them had had insufficient exposure to normal personal and social experiences. They displayed poor short-term memory and lacked physical coordination. They received training, care, and instruction—much of it contradictory—from a variety of caregivers. The result was they muddled what they might have mastered.

Many understood—as they stated in our group sessions—that they would require a lifelong support system. The significance of that was very real to them, and they took care not to alienate their caregivers. But independence is equally sweet to each one as to all of us, and each of us struggles to maintain what part of it we can manage alone. The ability to communicate insights varies from one person to another, and sometimes insight can be expressed without words. Whenever the personal consequences of an action are clear, we need not express our comprehension of it necessarily to feel it fully and possibly to change.

The core of the distress that attends a developmental disability often is a failure to acquire some amount of literacy. Considering how necessary it is to read in life, that handicap is a disaster. Encouragement to pursue different methods to obtain information and knowledge is important. When instruction and information are continuously available, continuous growth is achieved even though the pace may be slow. People thrive with respect and patience, and sometimes their dysfunction is in ratio to deprivations and subtle abuse. When the day comes that the whole population affected by mental retardation is offered lifetime learning opportunities, a greater normalcy will be possible for us all.

Reba, a middle-aged woman, was one client of the many from whom I learned; her story illustrates much of what can be typical among that group.[1] She and I were together for at least 10 years in work services. During that time, she helped me by providing authentic wisdom and by proffering a steady challenge to me to be as creative and transparent in my interactions with her as she was with me.

Reba had volunteered to lead all the workers in daily exercises in the cafeteria at break time. Together, she and I decided on the exercises, and we put pictures on cue cards. Even after 6 months of practice, she could not remember them consistently and would forget to look at her cards. Instead, delightfully, she would improvise. She would end the session on a comic note, and everyone would laugh and feel good. Reba enjoyed and accepted herself. She never thought she had to be perfect.

Reba also developed an effective vocabulary. One day in an occupational therapy group, I was showing a slide presentation that featured the Grand Canyon. I stumbled all over myself trying to explain in simple terms the differences between mountains and canyons. "It's scenery, Mildred, scenery," called out Reba, rescuing me and helping me to move on. I laugh and remember that day every time I complicate matters with too many words.

Reba's regular pastime was observing people. As she watched me work with others, she learned that my intention was to help clients accomplish tasks more easily. She tried to do the same for others, and she asked for help when a complex task needed to be divided into steps she could handle. When back trouble began to cause severe pain, she sought my help. I secured a chair and foot stool that supported her in a better postural alignment, and I had her practice some exercises. One winter, her tattered coat lost its last button. Reba waited for me to tell me about it. When we met, I offered to teach her how to sew the buttons back on, but she was not ready for that. "Not now, Mildred," was her diplomatic reply, and her eyes went to the sewing box in my open cabinet. I sewed as she watched.

Another time, however, her motivation moved her beyond the easy way out. At one group session, Reba enjoyed a new activity I had introduced that required holding two dowels in perpendicular fashion, one in each hand, to

---

[1]A version of the story about Reba originally appeared in my article "My Clients, My Mentors" in *Advance for Occupation Therapy*, October 4, 1999, and is adapted here with permission of *ADVANCE Newsmagazines*.

balance a horizontal dowel and roll it up and down with wrist action. Reba practiced a lot and became successful. The following week, she could do it better, and she squatted down, maintaining a straight, upright back, to pick up the horizontal dowel from the floor, spacing it perfectly across the two perpendicular dowels. How could she squat so well when she never had before? Previously she avoided bending because her girth made it troublesome. "I watched you," she said. She practiced the movement all week until my return. I had succeeded in piquing her interest, and now she was giving me good feedback. It was a reminder to me to relax and remember that people learn best when they perceive the need to acquire a skill.

Holding onto every moment of fun like a trolley hugging a track, Reba enhanced every group session. On one occasion, each member was given a chiffon scarf to use in movement exercises. Reba turned the scarf into a bridal veil and, hooking her arm into that of another member, she paraded around singing a wedding tune. Her example made the shy members feel safe enough to imitate her, and they did so with big smiles. Reba remembered some wedding ceremony rituals she could mimic. Her improvisations were hilarious.

Underneath Reba's actions was a desire to lead. However, sometimes her interactions in the group were unfair and other members would object. She needed to be persuaded to share and not to take extra turns, and she had to be reminded not to give help before it was wanted. With loud groans, she would protest the end of the sessions. However, to acknowledge her needs, I asked her to open the group session by shaking hands all around and then to initiate the exercises. Others could contribute, too. When the session was to end, Reba conducted closure, thanking everyone individually for coming and shaking hands again. She soon learned to be more aware of the feelings of others and to delay her own desires if she wanted the members to follow her lead.

Reba could cry at an offense, but she also could make a cool assessment. I remember when her longtime boyfriend left her for another woman. Reba took some time to absorb the infidelity, but within the hour, she turned back to her table and said, "Tomorrow he'll need me," and began talking with someone else. Practical and realistic, she looked to herself for positive comfort. I considered Reba my mentor; she was constantly teaching me so much. She and others, with all their differences, were treasures. Like the gems they were, they guided me into becoming more awake, more joyous, and more caring.

Methods and Treatment
in the Work Service Setting

When I began working at Goodwill Industries in the early 1980s, my clients mostly had moderate to profound impairments that could be addressed with adaptations. Their postures required improvement, or they needed assistance in sitting to reach for the items they used for work. Many needed treatment to strengthen or relax muscles or to increase the range of motion in their upper extremities. All corrections benefited their personal health and improved their productivity.

In one case, I worked closely with a physical therapist to provide care for Ellen, a client with paraplegia. Her legs needed stretching and strengthening, and she needed training in small motor skills. She had come to believe that she should use her hands only to use her special crutches. She had been relying on others for dressing and grooming, and she needed to learn to do those things for herself.

For treatment, the physical therapist helped her into a sitting position that had to be held for a prescribed period of time, and I supplied her with a hand-sewing project of her choice. That work occupied her while she sat for the required period. Over a time, the tasks were changed, and she began to use her hands to become independent in self-care. Ellen was in the high range of below-normal cognition, and part of her resistance to caring for herself was exhibited as belligerence toward staff members who had not been kind or understanding. When treated with respect, she responded very well. I learned from her what a difference a new approach can make when the client's acceptance is necessary. It was a pleasure to observe her striding along with increased confidence, clearly pleased with her attractive hairstyle, appropriate makeup, and stylishly crisp clothing.

Often the physical therapist would join me in conducting the five-stage session with the men and women in our clinic. He added greatly to my knowledge of good exercise, and I shared my understanding and assessments of the group members' visual, motor, or perceptual problems. We designed activities for the session to reduce the clients' difficulties and to encourage their abilities to emerge. This was a most productive period that reminded me of my past congenial collaborations with physical therapists. I was grateful for these second opportunities.

Once I asked the group members why they attended, and one client named Robert, who was easily agitated, answered in all seriousness, "To get rid of my aggravations!" So he benefited from the psychosocial aspects of the sessions as well as from the physical and motor-planning activities. The Five-Stage Group Model was appropriate for the setting because it gives comprehensive attention to practicing appropriate fine- and gross-motor movement. It allows every member an opportunity for spontaneous interaction, and it gives clients the same possibility for group engagement that is enjoyed by any other population.

In the workshop area, I explained to the supervisors that tasks could be broken down into simple parts that many clients could complete without help. At the time, clients were not allowed to work on a job unless they could finish unassisted. Even in the mid-1980s those approaches persisted, and they were coupled with a general disregard for the dignity of the employees. One supervisor told me that my example helped her to learn to address clients respectfully. She recognized that she received more cooperation when she did so. Her insight illustrates how surprised people are to learn how alike we all are in the way we respond to positive or negative behavior shown to us.

Renewing Clients Through Self-Achievement

In the latter part of the 1980s, I urged for the introduction of computers for workers. The agency liked the idea and at one point gave me an entire room for donated equipment. I had to vacate the area later when the space was needed for a new, faster moving program. One client was Bill, a middle-aged man with cerebral palsy that was marked by severe spasticity in all his extremities. Bill was barely able to vocalize and could not read beyond the first-grade level, yet he learned to use a computer by mastering a typing program with me called "Type to Learn." Despite his difficulty with spasticity, he was highly motivated and able to enter data by matching the shapes of letters. He lived at home and was proud that he could work on the computer just like his younger sister, who had a corporate job.

A local office of the Aetna insurance company had donated its 1970s-era computers to Goodwill. Bill helped me design written instructions using symbols and pictures for the especially lengthy routines required by the behemoth machines. One day I could not find the instructions. I was in a dither, fretting that I would need to write them all over again and, of course, blaming myself. When he was about to leave the clinic, Bill got my attention and vigorously pointed to a space below the table. I saw there a drawer I had not noticed before. It was natural in Goodwill to adapt donations like this table for use with the clients because funds for furniture were limited. Very little of the furniture we used was custom-designed for any particular use. I always was surprised to see how much of our discarded, donated items needed only imagination to become more functional.

Bill pointed to the paper with the rewritten instructions and again to the drawer. I understood, "Bill, you are wanting to organize me! You are right, we'll keep the instructions there, in YOUR drawer." His eyes lit up as he realized that I valued him. It was a splendid moment of connection for both of us because he was teaching me and he liked that. I was reminded that his great determination and cooperation had fired my intent to offer him my best during my dozen years with him.

In his middle years, his mother died. She was the linchpin in his physical care, and he realized a terrible loss. Although he showed a new inner strain as services and care for him lessened, I saw him rise as best he could to the circumstances at home and at work. When the moment he was living in was good, he appreciated it in a wonderful way, and his face glowed. He learned to revive himself in that way. A little compliment, a little attention, a small treat, a piece of work that came out well, a scarf placed around his neck for added warmth—all were renewing measures from which he drew deep pleasure.

That instructed and inspired me. Often we take for granted or ignore the small treats, attention, and unexpected brief pleasures that may occur to us that, if absorbed consciously, can refresh and renew us more than we may realize. I keep one of the small woven placemats that he made on a tiny two-harness loom to remind me of his intensity when doing his very best. Every one of his achievements made Bill proud. That was his great quality, and it helped him grow in self-enhancement.

Losing Funding

The Goodwill work service program in the early 1980s was considered a rehabilitation setting. In addition to the supervisory staff for the clients, the program consisted of a part-time physician, a part-time nurse, a full-time case manager, a part-time psychologist, a physical therapist, a speech therapist, and me. Several years before I departed in 1996, all of those people either had been discharged or had left without being replaced. Although I was the last remaining member of the rehabilitation staff, I failed to foresee the changes in the future of health care.

Grants and program renewals in earlier years had funded the salaries of rehabilitation workers. However, slowly reflecting a new philosophy emerging in state departments and other funding agencies, payments stopped. Programs either were dropped or scaled back because of reduced funding. In the past, when Goodwill had a full rehabilitation staff, that staff could help the needs and problems of the clients. With most of the staff now gone, house managers in the growing number of group homes were making major decisions for the clients living in the homes and were not relying on work placements like Goodwill to provide services. The house managers could decide to use other settings for psychology or physical therapy or take advantage of community resources to provide recreation or other services the residents required.

It was a microcosm of what was happening everywhere in health care. Gatekeepers determined which services were required, and decisions were being made by a new management with a new way to manage. Many people slipped through the cracks as different group homes operated under a variety of standards. And the profit motive entered in a new way in the work with people with chronic disabilities.

My world of work seemed intact, even as events around me showed grave changes. But as staffing continued to dwindle and employees were not replaced, as individual therapeutic programs were cut or abandoned, the changes began to affect me whether I was aware of it or not. My diversification clouded my view of conditions. Other contracts I held and liked, my research with Brenda Smaga, my writing and presenting of workshops— these held my interest. Sometimes a good friend would share a workshop with me. One such friend was Marcus Brown, PhD, a clinical psychologist. His interest in occupational therapy and his extensive knowledge in geriatrics and with groups made it natural for me to use his assistance and learn from him.

It finally happened that funding for my services was not forthcoming from the usual sources. Also, the activities that I could pursue were changing at Goodwill. The opportunity to work with groups was being curtailed, and I missed contact with my colleagues. As therapeutic programs for individual clients were discarded, the emphasis was on keeping clients busy whether or not the assigned tasks really produced cognitive or emotional gain. Often frustrated, the clients would become mischievous or destructive as they became bored or felt harassed. In 1996, I resigned with much regret and with great love for the population from whom I had learned and gained so much.

After leaving Goodwill, I began to pursue work in home care and on per diem contracts in other institutions. The events in the 1990s were affecting me. The spirit, mood, style, and needs of that decade necessarily brought change to everyone I knew.

chapter 6

THE 1990S:
HOME CARE

CHALLENGES TO HEALTH CARE
AND OCCUPATIONAL THERAPY

The 1990s began with troubling events held over from the 1980s, although things seemed to improve as the decade went by. A minor economic depression in the late 1980s got worse but then improved by the mid-1990s. Other events were important, too: The fall of the Berlin Wall in 1989 caused great elation. Desert Storm at the beginning of the decade was a mission that demonstrated our overall power to protect our interests. The end of the Cold War in 1992 reduced global tension. The success of Silicon Valley meant that technology was now front and center. The revived feeling of national safety was intoxicating, and a sense of individualism was renewed as more people experienced the value of their own competence (Padilla, 2005d). I continued to ignore how those events related to me, but whether or not I failed in awareness, occupational therapy was definitely affected.

The business side of health care was beginning to transfer into the hands of managed-care organizations that set out to control escalating costs and turn a profit. Early in the 1990s, the people spoke and rejected a universal health care policy that had promised to reduce administrative costs, one of the most expensive features in the new method of providing health care (Evanofski, 2003). The warning signs were loud and clear; yet independent, isolated service providers would continue work for some time before sounding the alarm for help from professional organizations. At first slowly, there began in the 1990s the end of generous opportunities in occupational therapy that had brought to the field a large supply of students and many job openings. So much was happening!

Reimbursements began to be limited, which would require state and national organizations to be vigilant to changes and respond to preserve services (Evanofski, 2003). Related professions then had to compete for access to limited resources. That required new methods of communication and negotiation among professions, like physical therapy, speech therapy, and occupational therapy that formerly had always collaborated. Staff reductions in hospitals, agencies, and long-term-care facilities provided growing evidence that there would be new ways to do business (Colmar, 1998; Diffendal, 1998; Steib, 1998). The expectation was that all service providers would need to examine their work to find ways to achieve more productivity by fewer people for less money. Experiencing the new upheaval, I observed many occupational therapists losing their positions. Educational programs closed. Smaller numbers of applicants enrolled in the remaining programs.

By the second half of the 1990s, the changes came more rapidly. The federal government withdrew as an assured payer for occupational therapists as Congress made drastic cuts to Medicare and Medicaid reimbursement (Evanoski, 2003). The rules tightened for use of occupational therapy in the rehabilitation process. Legislatures—federal and state—became increasingly indifferent to the idea of providing safety nets for disenfranchised populations: children, single parents, the terminally ill, people with mental health issues, and others. The reality was that the number of people who needed services was growing, and the number of services they needed was expanding as a larger percentage of the population became older and lived longer (Siebert, 2003). Would the poor, the old, and the stricken have to return to the largesse of the wealthy or to aid from religious institutions? Government action from the 1930s to the 1960s had turned away from those models. The 1970s and 1980s had seen even broader efforts and more progressive legislation. A guiding principle was being tested, and many issues in health care were being played out in the new Congress (Neistadt & Crepeau, 1998). The needs were the same as they had always been—if not even greater—but the perception of how to meet them had changed.

I view the 1990s as a decade strutting its scientific and technological gains, feeling confident in the political arena, but failing to value the good and generous advances for the disadvantaged that earlier decades had witnessed. The era offered drastic challenges to occupational therapists, who found grave changes in expectations. Those challenges spurred the profession on to new endeavors in practice. Home care and per diem work were two new opportunities. Even now, *OT Practice* magazine carries unusual, even brilliant, articles about private enterprise created by inventive occupational therapists.

When the decade ended, the unthinkable happened: The tragedy of September 11, 2001, brought a drastic awakening that at first created a national solidarity. It mobilized the best in our nation and demonstrated what good there always is in the undercurrent. We recognized more clearly that the reality of tragedy can be anyone's lot! Those who are injured will require all the different services in health care to recover. There is the need to watch lawmakers and what they are doing, encouraging them to be mindful of those who suffer great hardships. There is the need for all professionals to collaborate more, rather than to struggle for turf and self-gain, and for all citizens to collectively do more vocalizing and voting.

The basic human needs we have been accustomed to serve are still here. New ways for occupational therapy to flourish with new ideas, in new places, and with new skills arise from the inevitability of change and from the general suffering that includes poverty, disability, and low expectations seen around us. Occupational therapists now in graduate school will be ready to meet the new demands, but they must be abundantly resourceful to uphold the profession.

Sharing Knowledge Through Publishing

In the 1990s, my first three books went out of print, and I regained their copyrights. One day in 1994, I visited Marilyn Cole, a longtime friend and the author of *Group Dynamics in Occupational Therapy* (1998). Marilyn is an experienced teacher and scholar, and occupational therapy students everywhere use her text. In 2007, she became Professor Emeritus at Quinnipiac University. When our conversation turned to my writing and how to renew it she astonished me by speedily providing a list of options I should consider. Suggesting another publisher might be interested in a revision of one book, she added three other themes about which she believed I could write. One can see how she brought out the best in students; she certainly ignited my motivation. Sitting with the right person, an understanding and creative friend, helped me. Less than a decade later, the American Occupational Therapy Association (AOTA) honored her contributions to the discipline when it named her a Fellow.

I did follow her advice. In 1997 AOTA Press published *Integrative Group Therapy: Mobilizing Coping Abilities with the Five-Stage Group.* Then, in 1998, Susan Bachner, MS, OTR/L, FAOTA, CEAC, and I collaborated on *Adults with Developmental Disabilities: Current Approaches in Occupational Therapy.* Susan has outstanding expertise in the subject after almost 40 years of clinical practice. In watching her work with this special population, I saw her insight, imagination, and interest bring out their best. She has expanded her knowledge by obtaining credentials in environmental consulting, and she guides the transformation of inaccessible and unsafe residences into supportive environments or consults on new related projects. Susan and I revised and updated our book in 2004.

There have been many changes in publishing since my first entry in 1981. Now there are tougher standards, as publishers must consider the risks of publishing any book. A publisher once explained to me that he was willing to accept manuscripts that might not be best sellers because he wanted to have a well-rounded inventory. Now, the marketplace is too complicated to rely on a publisher's personal belief that subject matter is as important as whether a book will sell. Nevertheless, there is a market for good work, and persistence pays.

Working With Clients in Home Care

Ingenuity and good judgment are essential for home care practice, and the setting holds the possibility for occupational therapists to contribute, in collaboration with caregivers and clients, to a realistic support system for the client. This was the principle it held for me. Every home has a unique culture. Expectations differ widely for what constitute cleanliness, organization, activities of daily living (ADLs), food appreciation and preparation, connected relationships, use of leisure time, or locus of control. All of those areas are affected for someone who must now learn new ways to retain essential functions following illness or disability, and each of them requires thoughtful consideration from the occupational therapist. Home care is difficult work. A visit may demand more time than is generally available, and there is a great temptation to attempt to work on too many issues at once. Trying to reconcile all the elements involved to achieve the safest and most beneficial outcome for the client can be daunting. However, learning to confine treatment to what is immediately manageable is the best place to start; resolution of the referral issue first can help other issues fall in place for a longer term plan.

During the 1980s and 1990s, my private practice included several home care contracts. They tested my ingenuity, self-confidence, and moral judgment. I learned that a sense of humor was crucial, and that humor always could be found in the midst of serious issues and difficulties. The story of one of my first home care visits is a case in point. During a homemaking session, and much to my astonishment, a client cut a head of cabbage *in mid-air* before I could do anything to stop her. The workspace in her kitchen had forced her to develop this dangerous adaptation.

The same client required shoulder strengthening (although I wondered about that as I caught her work with the head of cabbage), so I provided a game called "The Frog Catches the Fly," which would require the use of her shoulder muscles. I was impressed that she seemed to enjoy a little challenge with some playfulness. The object of the game is to trap a marble that is connected by a string to a wooden clapper. The clapper was attached to the client's palm, and as the client swung her arm she tried to close the clapper to catch the fly (marble). At first her shoulder movements were too feeble for her to swing the marble out and pull it back, but she persisted for about three weeks until she achieved a good degree of strength and progress—as well as delight with her success. We also uncovered some counter space in her tiny kitchen so that she could cut vegetables or anything else comfortably and safely on a countertop and no longer work in the air.

Sometimes staggering difficulties in the home can seem almost unreal, even comical. One asks, "What else can happen here?" Another of my first contacts was Angela, a young woman who had to wear a heavy halo brace as part of the treatment for a cervical spine condition she had developed from a parasite infection contracted in South America. Angela shared a fourth-floor walkup in a tenement apartment house with her active seven-year-old son and her frail but overprotective mother. Issues with finances, transportation, and language barriers were among her other challenges. Her physician's referral to me consisted of orders to strengthen her upper arms and back. We rearranged the kitchen to meet her presenting limitations, worked on various crafts that she also could use with her son, and discussed how her mother might help in a collaborative way without overdoing. Angela made a macramé belt for her son as one craft both could learn. Macramé can be graded to be easy work or positioned to produce greater resistance for appropriate muscle strengthening. I saw her courage in meeting a multitude of problems during her progress. Remarkably, she was able to laugh when the brace finally was removed and I identified with her joy.

Astonishment sometimes leads to humor when an unsuspected talent emerges in a client. Chloe had Down syndrome and had been diagnosed with depression. She lived independently, and her referral was for help in improving her homemaking skills. We wrote down recipes of dishes that we cooked together. This led to organizing shopping lists and to choosing the kinds of foods that would help her lose weight. She also needed signs and labels to help her organize her laundry, to remind her to change vacuum cleaner bags, or to point out safety and cleanliness issues. The signs helped her to remember not to stack cereal boxes or loaves of bread on the floor when she ran out of pantry space.

Although Chloe seemed to listen to instructions, she paid them scant attention. Chloe had a conservator who had shared her frustration with me about Chloe's unconventional behaviors. At the end, I saw that Chloe managed better by being less dogmatic than I was about how things should be done. I requested and received extended visits to her and finally concluded that she had achieved an acceptable standard for safety.

It had been a conundrum for me that Chloe exhibited considerable talent as an artist. She created lively and orderly paintings, yet she could not learn to put her untidy room in order. I concluded that for some matters she always would require supervision, direction, and physical assistance, and this would have to be arranged. When I reported this, her conservator agreed, and Chloe continued to live independently. On my last day with her, she surprised me again. As we took leave of each other, she reached for her camera and asked me to stand by the light at the door while she snapped a picture of me for her scrapbook. I think of Chloe and feel she had a blithe spirit that was endearing and memorable. She discovered that producing surprise and playfulness helped her more than being spic and span.

In the end, I concluded that Chloe had sufficient awareness of her health and her relationships but that she was satisfied with much less than those who supervised her could be. She had a sense of contentment and self-acceptance, but she also had the ability to recognize when she needed to seek help. All of that contributed to her emotional well-being, and that in turn permitted her to live independently, which she prized. I learned from her about being open to more flexible criteria for independent living.

Sometimes the beautiful spirit of a client lights up the environment with an unexpected cheerfulness, faith, and a quiet acceptance, despite grim circumstances. Mr. Franklin was an elderly client who lived alone in a renovated apartment in an old school building. He had moderate asthma and had had an above-the-knee amputation of his left leg. He refused to wear his artificial limb, preferring to use his wheelchair for mobility. He wanted an electric wheelchair. He was slender and agile and would park his chair outside the bathroom door and leap over the sink to the toilet. I persuaded him that it would be safer, although less dramatic, to take his wheelchair into the bathroom so he could transfer more safely to the commode. The new method disappointed him, I think, because it lacked imagination. Still, he accepted it when we practiced this.

During my visits, we went down to the street so I could appraise his ability to go a distance and cross a street safely. It became apparent he was heedless of safety, and he was inclined to overestimate his endurance: As he went longer distances he showed he did not have the stamina he needed for return trips. Without daily prompting, he would not do the exercises prescribed to maintain flexibility. He accepted that assessment with good grace, in keeping with his personality. It was his way to accept whatever the day presented. I admit it was fun to be with him because of his cheerfulness. He seemed to think he ought to entertain me, and it was interesting to hear his dramatic stories of his days out west. His spirit refused to be dampened. He was a great talker who reminded me of a favorite uncle. I suffered a loss when the visits ended, but I recognized that he inspired acceptance of life's daily challenges.

Dealing With Marital Discord

There was little humor in the home of a couple in their late 80s who were trying hard to retain control over their life together—and to be polite about it. The husband had a stroke at the same time the wife was returning home from hospitalization for a liver ailment. Both of them had to keep track of visits from nurses, aides, and physical and occupational therapists. I was assigned to provide a general assessment of ADLs, physical functioning, and cognitive functioning. The husband had been mildly affected by the stroke, and both he and his wife required overall strengthening and assistance with modifications and adaptive equipment.

On the first visit, the husband requested help from me to understand the bills, Medicare, and hospital notices that were troubling him. This concern was primary to him and in a few visits was brought under control. However, I was aware of another, larger problem. The couple was overwhelmed by the staggering and exhausting number of visits from health care staff. I did not believe I was of minimal use, but in the general context of what was a priority, the other visiting staff were being put to good use. I expressed that assessment to the agency. I believed that, given time, the outcomes this stressed couple required could be achieved without me. It seemed as though they were getting too much of too many good things, and someone had to make this decision. I felt satisfied at their obvious relief and the knowledge that they had one another and plenty of other supports, at least for the immediate term.

In an earlier time, I visited a home in a small manufacturing town. The husband was house bound, and his middle-aged wife took care of him. Mr. Black had been a bricklayer who had sustained a recent terrible fall that resulted in injury to his cervical area, requiring almost total assistance in all ADLs. He was making some improvement, but very slowly.

My referral directed that I find some way in which Mr. Black might use his small amount of active movement in the upper right extremity to feed himself. The visit was assigned to me in the early 1980s, before many of the current inventive measures for self-feeding were available. I worked on strengthening what I could with touching, moving, and facilitating his upper extremity. Mr. Black was positioned in a wheelchair with supports for sitting upright and receiving assistance for getting ready for the day from an aide who came each morning to help his wife. During my visit and my exploratory trials with devices and palm cuffs, Mr. and Mrs. Black discussed with me the kinds of foods that made eating easier, diversions that might be introduced, and an array of concerns around Mr. Black's weakened condition. Those conversations were not easy to sustain; I had an intuition that Mrs. Black wanted to just deliver the minimum service necessary without extending any more. She was aloof and cool to Mr. Black, who spoke almost exclusively to me. Mrs. Black was in the extraordinary position of having great demands placed upon her while Mr. Black seemed stoic in his tolerance of his circumstances, but it seemed that he took his wife's service for granted.

Even now, I am uneasy about exploring the serious picture of the lack of any kind of personal warmth in that home. I began to develop some understanding when, alone with Mrs. Black by chance, she indicated to me that her marriage had been bleak and that her husband was a harsh man who had not been attentive to her in earlier years. I wondered how all this was going to play out when more recovery was achieved. Deciding to stay within the realm of what was expected of me, I suggested to Mrs. Black the need to talk about her feelings in counseling sessions outside the home. She was not interested. I never brought it up again.

As I continued to help Mr. Black to learn to eat independently and to perform some ADLs, he began to flirt with me. He could not reach out, so he began to form kisses with his lips and throw them to me. Under the circumstances, this easily could be ignored. In general, the home presented a barren atmosphere both physically and emotionally. Here was a woman who was living in anger with her previously robust husband, who now expressed liveliness in the only way he could. I had just a few more visits before my work was completed. Telling him this, I ignored his behavior. I wish now I had boldly advised him to turn his charms toward his wife, but I missed that chance. I even could have reinforced that a smile, a "please," or a "thank you" would help. When he blew me kisses at our last meeting, I smiled because his wife happened to come into the room just at that time. I made a departure statement wishing them good luck, and I warmly touched the shoulders of both.

My early professional training promoted the reserve in my behavior that took time to modify with some graciousness and common sense. However, thinking of this couple and how I might have changed my behavior in order to modify theirs, I wished they had been able to learn, as I had, that a little playfulness goes a long way to lighten dreary routine and misgivings. That was something that my dear Chloe understood so easily. Support for both partners required strengthening of spirit as much as strengthening Mr. Black's muscles.

Another case provided a nearly opposite situation. The wife of a retired couple was returning from a serious hospitalization and needed to use a wheelchair. Although her husband seemed able-bodied to me, he had been accustomed to his wife's waiting on him in his new period of retirement. Now, she was unable to cook, and for several weeks after her discharge, neighbors sent meals in or the couple ate frozen dinners.

Mr. Clark complained bitterly about this. My referral was to assess the wife's ability to resume some of her previous tasks in the kitchen. Mrs. Clark had full use of her hands and arms, and she appeared neat in her attire, but she seemed timid in her behavior. The home and kitchen were tidy. I asked Mrs. Clark how she had prepared a meal before her hospitalization. She described the way she gathered what she needed, carried the supplies to the table, and stood there to prepare the meal. I assured her that the same method could be used, only now she could do her preparation sitting. Mrs. Clark required the assurance that sitting while preparing food was an acceptable method and quite possible. Occupational therapists reframe situations consciously and unconsciously as a matter of course, but habits and routines can clog the process for those who resist new methods.

Mr. Clark was instructed in providing a rolling cart that his wife could use for food preparation. Fortunately, Mrs. Clark found the table to be a good height for preparation, but the use of the refrigerator and stove also had to be assessed. Mr. Clark would now need to help more than had been his habit, and he showed his disappointment at the new turn of events. How could he become the support his wife required?

Quite often marital discord was the undercurrent of my home visits. It was like a pile of overlooked or hidden agendas, and it definitely hindered progress. Often, there is grumbling, "I would like to leave." Unlike the circumstances of my clients Diane or Sally, where the sweetness of family strength and support were evident, illness in the stories of the Blacks and the Clarks exacerbated an already unpleasant situation.

I believed I was unqualified to explore or analyze those relationships. Nothing in my schooling and little in the literature related to an occupational therapist's role in such circumstances. I became more aware of the sad fact that those unhappy relationships were more common than I had believed, and I began to consider the need to do something about it as I met it in home care. The issue was whether I should ignore the crumbling remains of a deteriorated relationship, refer to it directly by advising outside counseling, or try to see how to help each mate appreciate the other's value without obviously extolling either one excessively. I believe there must be other methods to explore. I think this area could be a fruitful one to examine in the classroom; I wish I had been able to learn more about how to cope with it before I had to confront it.

Mr. Clark represents any number of the spouses I met in home care. They did not hide their disappointment with their mates' inability to provide a service they believed was an entitlement, and they were not reluctant to share any grievance. The subject of relationships is personal and complex. In the Clarks' case, I decided to energize the husband to encourage him to rise to the situation. I did that by articulating the problems his wife had demonstrated, and then I waited to see what solution he would find. It was interesting that he could shop for groceries, so long as his wife wrote out a list. He could adapt the stove to her needs, and he could rearrange some of the kitchen equipment to help her manage better.

Mrs. Clark and I both gave him a lot of praise for his effort. The larger picture of a more satisfying relationship went unfulfilled. There was more involved than simply making meals. Because I was seeing the same problems in so many homes, I wondered whether I could come better armed by declaring openly that "a sudden, terrible illness can turn a marriage upside down." I could add that if this were true for either partner, there are competent providers who can offer hope and lead the partners to clarity on the situation. I could carry with me the names of organizations to suggest.

I believe the home care assignments helped me to understand that marriages do not always fail because of the sudden calamity of illness. A necessary part of healing, for the whole situation, could be the mending of the underlying discontent and of coming to an understanding of how the illness might have and could now be used to bring more wellness into family life. Whatever the therapist is comfortable with ought to be tried so that the situation is not ignored. Providing a referral to an appropriate counselor might be the best route, and it helps fill out the necessary support system that, as I stated in the beginning of this chapter, can be a principle for initiating home care. One learning experience for me was that it is important at least to recognize and to come to some decision about acting on a recurring, underlying problem. I would not have ignored it so totally as I had.

MENTAL HEALTH ISSUES IN HOME CARE

Home care practice for people with physical disabilities had for several decades been a customary service. However, home health care for those with mental or behavioral health issues was slow to arrive in Connecticut and became generally available only in the 1990s. In 1996, I contracted with a home health agency for the first time to treat clients recently discharged from psychiatric settings. Some of the identified needs of those clients included time or budget management, homemaking skills, safety, transportation, caregivers' concerns, and the use of social or leisure skills. My hourly assignment included transportation time and a probable call to a medical supply house for equipment or to the social services department for permission to order that equipment. The client's doctor or nurse often required a call to verify or guide my decision. The documentation included as briefly as possible all the actions taken. Usually, all goals were expected to be achieved within a specific period, often just 9 to 12 visits.

Although time consuming, describing occupational therapy to the nurses in the agency was necessary because my referrals came chiefly from them. I admired and appreciated the life-giving care nurses provided, and I explained how I could enhance a program for specific clients. Often we worked out creative solutions to problems; for example, for persons diagnosed with dementia or for those who had both behavioral health issues and physical disabilities. I enjoyed the noncompetitive, mutually respectful atmosphere in the agency where I worked.

Among my first agency referrals was Holly, a young woman diagnosed with obsessive–compulsive disorder (OCD), a condition that seriously interfered with her daily functioning. After several psychiatric hospitalizations, Holly was living in a three-room apartment, which was considered a more economical way for the state to provide for her care. Her showers would take 4 hours or more, and that made her late for medical or other appointments. Her diet of fast food left her kitchen counters littered with piles of cartons and leftover food that was never placed in the refrigerator or put out with the trash. Her closets and drawers were empty because all of her clothing, clean and dirty, was in heaps on the bedroom floor with her other belongings. She explained to me that beginning any activity overwhelmed her, and she would sit on her couch for hours waiting to become moved to act, even though that never happened.

Holly was a pretty woman with abundant wavy hair, slender and graceful in her movements. During one of my earliest visits, a handsome young man had come during his lunch hour to drop off a bag of quarters for Holly to use in the building's laundry room. She told me that they had been dating regularly, most recently attending a sports event. They had had a giggling good time, racing up the concrete stairs to the highest level in the stadium. Holly expressed her pleasure at attention from the opposite sex and of having a good time. She also expressed a longing for meaningful ways to spend her time.

From Holly I came to understand the vastness of the illness, of the strength of the compulsions that can control a life. I also came to learn my limits. Despite my intentions, my strong interest, and my careful discussions with her about her expressed needs, I learned that if it came to a choice between an obsessive or compulsive behavior and an important desire or opportunity, her choice was to drop the desire or opportunity.

About a year later, I learned more while at work on a hospital ward where several patients diagnosed with OCD received treatment. I saw their pain and the difficulty with treatment, but also I witnessed the triumph of some victory. OCD treatment was intense and coordinated, continuously monitored by ward staff. Patients received medication and followed individually designed programs that used a "fading-out" conditioning to help them accept healthier behaviors. They were expected to attend group therapy as well as other scheduled appointments throughout the day. The ward had the rigor of a boot camp.

Holly's condition never did subside. Her young man became discouraged and disappeared as others had in the past. Her nurse complained about Holly's constant lack of compliance or inability to take medication consistently. I found that Holly's caseworker was completely disillusioned about the possibility of any progress, although she did grant my request for more time. I used collaborative work with Holly as she chose tasks like sorting laundry, organizing possessions, creating a scrapbook of her writing and items of interest, and cooking meals. Once she even invited company for a meal and reported how much it was enjoyed. We tried to concoct a variety of boundaries to limit her obsessive behaviors. For exercise, we ran together up and down the staircases in her apartment house. In the end, Holly chose to accept her illness and decided to ask for a home health aide to clean her apartment. Her request was granted because the unsanitary conditions otherwise would have presented a hardship for her neighbors.

Holly's illness had begun in her preadolescence, and her condition had worsened as she aged. She was always forthright in our discussions during our work together. She demonstrated grave difficulty, for example, with sorting laundry: For her, it meant making tiny piles of clothing, all to be washed separately. The task took hours to complete and many quarters.

Over time we were able to negotiate what seemed to be an agreeable middle ground. But it was not really agreement. Rather, she hoped that something miraculously would make her better. She never completely accepted that there could be a connection between performing an activity and gaining a more normal way of spending time. She could not follow any routine we established unless I was there. This does demonstrate that, in order to change, the person who is ill must verbalize the desire to change and have a goal in mind. The client must have the strength of conviction that change is possible, despite the work involved. Otherwise, treatment results can be dismal.

The only hope for Holly would have been a support system that imposed a structured and supervised daily arrangement of workers visiting her, taking turns motivating her, and checking on her progress. Compliance with medication, for example, could have been a crucial step for Holly because compliance is a first step in the schedule of daily activities. Imposed, habitual, daily practice might have reduced her anxieties and could possibly have helped her overcome her need to express her power in a useless manner. Holly was unable to take advantage of the large amount of assistance she was receiving because she required daily supervision, and home care does not supply this. A team approach and daily group therapy appear to bring more success with OCD.

Mary was a good example for me of how much society's attitude toward caring for those with mental health disorders has changed over the decades. Mary lived on her own on the third floor, formerly the attic, of a renovated old house. She was very similar to people I once had been accustomed to seeing on the large day wards in the state psychiatric hospitals where, indeed, she had spent many years. In her early 50s, she was known for her explosive, unpredictable behavior, and she exhibited an overall slight tremor, very visible around her mouth, which had been caused by long-term use of certain psychotropic drugs.

Mary was overweight, and although she generally appeared cleanly attired, she was a bit disheveled overall. She experienced mood swings and the effects of schizophrenia, which was the basis for her sometimes confused and resistive response to even small changes. She was sometimes self-destructive in terms of her diet and smoking; going out to strange, possibly unsafe places; and occasionally throwing large objects, including pieces of furniture, out of her window. All the same, she had a charismatic side, and all of her providers consistently were devoted to her welfare. She demonstrated a core of vibrancy that had survived her years with an oppressive illness. Those qualities were clear in her conversations, which could be unpredictably funny or suddenly very astute. Sometimes, unexpectedly, she would follow a suggestion. She had an undeniable charm. She was living with greater independence now than would have been considered possible in previous decades.

Mary's social contact came chiefly from a devoted social worker and a home health aide faithfully involved in her care. A nurse who visited her regularly had referred me because she was concerned that Mary was unsafe in her bathroom. The bathtub was a freestanding model, and there was nothing for Mary to hold onto as she climbed in. The corner of the bathroom had a tiny sink, in which Mary insisted that the aide wash her hair. She refused to allow the nurse to watch her bathing to assess her safety. I knew that social services would not pay for a grab bar over the tub because such an appliance was considered unsafe, as it has been known to slip.

I asked Mary to get into the tub fully dressed to show me her ordinary method. She complied with ease and did so safely. She accepted a hand-held shower that I got installed so she could wash her own hair, and she accepted a tub mat and a nonslip throw rug next to the tub. The nurse and I were satisfied with the results.

The lighting in Mary's kitchen was configured so that her body created a shadow that forced her to work in the dark at the stove and at the sink. I arranged better lighting, and the aide used nail polish to mark the stove knobs for visibility. Additional safety measures, like removing the bottle of cooking oil kept on the stove and adding reminder lists and tools for cleaning methods, were provided.

When Mary complained of a backache, I checked on her bedding. I found that her mattress had split in two and the bedsprings were worn out. The agency's staff secured new bedding. In addition to other suggestions on activities, I thought to tempt her with some colorful books on interesting subjects. We talked about them, but her motivation was not strong enough for her to continue on her own when I would not be with her. My hope was that in the future another occupational therapist would be called on to assist Mary.

Because Mary was feisty and challenged any suggestion, I worked with her lack of trust by being sure to get her agreement with each step I took. At this time, she did not need to have the door locked behind her by others; she was able to lock her door after the visits of concerned and trained workers. For as long as her safety continued, I was glad to see that the solution was to allow her greater independence but to maintain needed supports. That approach was far better for people like Mary than the institutionalization that would have been required in an earlier time. Mary's life was very much enhanced by the good attentions she received from the agency workers; that was no accident, as she attracted much interest from others. Society deserves a notch up for Mary's greater freedom.

I resigned my home care position when I contracted with a psychiatric hospital in 1997 for a per diem arrangement so that my time would become better structured during the working day.

chapter 7

REFLECTION

The work of a lifetime that one does is a significant factor in the later years. Therefore, instead of separating work from other parts of our life it is beneficial to tie it all together. Whatever is learned in a job practiced with passion, truth, fairness, best endeavor, and patience can be carried over into our private life and, of course, the other way around. Occupational therapy practice is rich in this way. We are not looking for perfection but for integration in our behavior.

For example, I began to see that what I said to the people I treated was different from what I practiced myself. I would decide on goals that I needed to achieve and then make choices that could never lead to the outcomes I desired. I would never counsel any-one else to do that. It was about midway through my career, in the late 1970s, that I began to feel strongly that I wanted to prac-tice what I talked about with others. I would treat myself to more of everything like thoughtful choices, self-discipline, generosity, and self-acceptance. If a pattern of daily routine—good nutrition, mental and physical exercise, and meditation—was beneficial for the people I treated, why not for me? It is easy to appreciate that the aspiration is simple but maintaining the regimen is harder!

As an example of this, I return to a home care assignment where I was referred to a client in behavioral health to work on budget management. She spent about half of her very small income on cigarettes. We explored how to modify this behavior, but it made me reflect on my own indulgences and how I could work to put my own house in order. I quickly was reminded of the difficulty of reining in my own habits of quick gratification. As I did this while working with her, it gave me the compassion to understand her even though I had so little in common with her addiction. Often we think we have understanding and compassion, but it is not until we are faced with the same need to be understood that we learn more about those qualities.

The small state psychiatric hospital I joined when I gave up my home care assignments provided increased learning experiences. I worked for the first time with substance abuse patients with and without psychosis and with patients who had known chronic emotional illnesses that included obsessive–compulsive disorder (OCD), bipolar disorder, and schizophrenia.

As I planned group work on renewing or creating healthy lifestyles, I also took them to heart and thought about them realistically. I hoped and expected that the group members would participate as I listened carefully to their responses and chose themes to introduce that would motivate them to design their own healthy lifestyles.

The group members I treated, despite their chronic illnesses, had a good level of cognition. I decided that I could upgrade the Five-Stage Group Model I had created for populations that were more behaviorally and cognitively challenged. My new clients needed the same approach of being eased into a group's session; most of them did not want to believe they belonged in the hospital. This meant they would benefit from a slow and friendly start at the beginning of the group session. Each meeting began with a personal acknowledgment of each participant and an examination of some curiosity that I introduced. Time would always be taken for active movement, whether with weights or Thera-Band elastic strips for resistive exercise, batons or scarves for aerobics, and so on.

The members of the group were educated in public schools; all of them could read and write, and some had college degrees. I could introduce, therefore, more challenging tasks within each stage, such as worksheets with instructions for testing perceptual or cognitive skills, that would not have been possible for some of my earlier groups of clients. The goals for group members were to learn something useful and to feel recharged and calm when the session ended. What I was most pleased with was that, in using the five stages, we would make time to use appropriate exercise, which is so important in behavioral health. In most centers, clients can be left to sit, slumped and listless, for long periods.

Generally, although everyone participated willingly in the exercises, some members did not enjoy my themes for their cognitive tasks. I was surprised to find a lack of enthusiasm for a discussion about the inspiration we can take from our culture's role models. Many of the group members had scant knowledge about heroes from history or literature or about others to whom society is indebted—even when I brought in pictures or showed films. And if the members were familiar with those people, the history seemed to have little relevance for their lives. Some members, however, saved the day when they sang the praises of a parent or other relative, a teacher, or a friend. Their inspiration needed to come from personal experience, and I learned from this.

Another theme I introduced that did not get a standing ovation from the group was the idea of organizing their daily routines. As I handed each member a notebook to use to keep track of items to buy, tasks to complete, or ideas for a journal, I had to offer many examples of how to make lists; it was difficult for them to organize their thoughts in those areas. And the idea of learning how to tie a necktie, sew a button, or fix a hem made their eyes glaze over! However, whenever I gave members 15 minutes to write a poem, there was great enthusiasm and willing compliance. The members expressed their feelings of pain, resignation, or gratitude. Few expressed reluctance to engage in this task and mostly the results were offered with pride. I thought about this and realized that the group members were in the throes of angst and addressing that pain was their priority. This they could do with poetry. Although I was sympathetic, I also considered that often there are concrete chores that need to be accomplished in a normal day. I continued to offer that more practical and applied direction too, and I worked at thinking of palatable ways to do so.

It is clear that there were many challenges in offering therapeutic group activities to the people on this ward. Each client was expected to attend every session offered. The groups were not homogeneous in age, diagnosis, ability, or life experience. One member might have a doctorate, another could be a homeless person who had not completed high school, and a third might have a diagnosis of Down syndrome.

It became clear to me how mental pain, equal to any physical pain, fills the heart and mind of the person with an emotional illness. I never forgot this when understanding behavior and responding to it. A group member described this distress in his poem:

> MY MIND
> *My mind is a raging river. Full of strong currents.*
> *Troubled waters, a never-ending flow of torment.*
> *My mind is like a sick river flooding over the banks, out of control.*
> *I feel as though I'm drowning.*
> *I pray some day this loud river will turn into a gentle stream.*

John, another group member, was a client diagnosed with OCD. He was well-educated—he had a doctorate—but he was unable to function at home or at work because of his compulsive behaviors. I always had his attention; he needed to participate so he could greet my suggestions with scorn. One day in the late 1990s, I was giving an overview on meditation. Many group members found the idea difficult to accept, although a few said they were willing to try. I told them that the physical changes during meditation could bring their bodies to a state of relaxation that could lead to a reduction in anxiety and emotional distress and thus improve physical health. John said, "Isn't it true Mildred, that sexual intercourse offers the best opportunity to feel relaxed?" John had not meant it to be, but that remark was an act of kindness. The pause that followed allowed everyone to focus their attention on me, and that gave me the opportunity to redirect the group in a productive way. "John," I said, as I took my time to fix my attention on him, "You are right." Then I added, "However, sometimes we lack the opportunity. I am showing the group another way to relax." I returned to my subject.

I think that small episode helped defuse the trepidation some members felt about the subject of meditation. Because the tension seemed reduced and attention was focused as I had wanted it to be, John had helped everyone. When we began the exercise, time was allotted for the participants to close their eyes and sit silently. One young woman appeared especially moved. In the discussion that followed she said, "This is the first time I ever had permission or took the time to concentrate on me!" Within a group, the therapist deals with all degrees of resistance and needs to balance what appears to be required so that most of the members will be served.

There were other occasions when John tried to disrupt a session. It was clear to me that he was troubled, pained, and conflicted; making cynical remarks was an outlet for him. One day, however, a young woman who had a developmental disability appropriately devised a simple, impromptu game of toss. To support her, John took up her task with gusto so she would succeed. I was moved by his gracious behavior, and it might have been a turning point for him as he began to extend himself, putting aside some of his self-absorption.

Sometimes it is in a group session that a therapist can recall the sudden, positive change that marks the beginning of recovery for a client. Earlier I recounted the story of one of my first groups at Connecticut Valley Hospital, when one group member became angry with me at my unexpected touch. Then, a few days later, she was discharged because she had found her voice. Three or four weeks after this event, John had improved so much that he was discharged home to his wife and children. On the day he left, he gave me a hug and thanked me for my patience. He had come a long way from believing he would contaminate others with toxins if he touched them.

The groups I treated in that last placement were the most diverse of my experience. That diversity in itself can hamper cohesiveness and impede bonding. Still, I saw on many occasions that the innate goodness in people emerges even during their worst times. Often, I could use the abilities of the stronger, the smarter, the more understanding to reach out and give help to those less well endowed. I tried to create those opportunities. In that way, at least, the lack of group homogeneity became an asset.

It was difficult to leave the setting. I was learning so much, but my hearing was deteriorating. Team meetings with other staff members and larger group sessions were becoming more difficult for me as I failed to hear soft speech or the quick asides that go on among people. It was necessary for me to resign in 1998.

"As we do so we become."
—David Nelson
Eleanor Clarke Slagle Lecture, 1996

The practice of occupational therapy has changed substantially since 1950, although the qualities required by therapists remain the same. As Suzanne M. Peloquin (2005) said in "Embracing Our Ethos, Reclaiming Our Heart," her Eleanor Clarke Slagle Lecture,

When, in spite of constraints, practitioners make their interventions meaningful, lively, and even fun, they infuse therapy's purposive aims with its capacity to encourage and inspire. Acting on the belief that occupation fosters dignity, competence, and health, we embrace the spirit of the profession. As we enable healing occupations, we reclaim our heart. (p. 623)

The practice will continue to change in response to a changing society's needs and prevailing spirit. We will continue to address new research and the results of discoveries in medicine and technology. Some of the new domains of concern for occupational therapists include working with populations that suffer the results of natural and human-made disasters, terrorism, global warming, HIV/AIDS, domestic abuse, homelessness, and increased longevity. There is a necessity for intervention in those areas because of the resulting terrible physical and emotional consequences for people throughout the world.

One obvious conclusion from this review of the past is that events and people constantly are in flux, changing for better or for worse. We tend to take for granted how life appears right now to us and to ignore gradual or dramatic change. As changes occur, whether beneficial or not, they may be disregarded or responded to with a sense of helplessness. When necessary action is delayed, we do not consider what values, conditions, or beliefs we may be perpetuating that we do not want and eventually will have to struggle with undoing. However, sometimes change is bracing!

The need to embrace change can be observed in the progress of the development of occupational therapy. This is seen as we enlarge our scope in every direction: in the science of occupation, in expanding treatment for behavioral or physical trauma, in exploring spirituality, and in research and writing. A master's degree is now a professional requirement, and it provides equality in credentials to peer professions.

I have used my own questions to assess the personal value of the years of endeavor in this profession and have used the narratives to provide the answers. Such questions remain an individual matter. How much satisfaction did I achieve, and what was its origin? How can I express my gratitude for the profound help and guidance I received from family, clients, teachers, friends, and mentors? What were the outcomes of the changes that occurred in every area during the working years? Were they challenges I was prepared to meet? Where did I find opportunities to stay informed and updated? Could I be kept completely absorbed in some part of the work? How were personal beliefs and values managed throughout the time of work? Do I feel increased energy, satisfaction, and interest from the work that comes my way, be it in practice, study, or writing?

Appreciating the connection I could make with clients often gave me a sense of complete absorption in the practice. Related to this was the availability of additional knowledge and expertise throughout my career that was provided by the state; by my other employers; and by other professionals, including the physicians, nurses, psychologists, and physical and occupational therapists who readily shared their knowledge in workshops or privately. I easily adopted an attitude of acceptance toward beginning anew, as I often had to do. The additional knowledge I acquired made me ready to address new opportunities that arose, as they surely always did, when I tapped into the resources of each new work environment.

Whenever I saw the indomitable spirit of a person emerge from his or her struggle to heal, I felt inspired and gratified. I saw new heroes. It took an elderly woman who had severe arthritis and was recovering from hip surgery three long weeks to master the equipment I provided her to put on her socks. But the day came that she did not need the equipment, and when she could succeed without it, she swept me along with her victory. The preacher, recovering from a stroke with a permanently left flaccid arm, worked hard to regain the ability to shine his own shoes. I demonstrated the technique for him, and he mastered it. That showed how important it was for his spirit, and he later gave me an audiotape of his powerful and passionately delivered sermons. I surmised that he believed that even his shoes should reflect the fervor and passion of his message. His goals guided his actions, and he returned to the pulpit.

I had exceptional mentors and teachers who took the time to help shape my beliefs and actions. During my internship at the Veterans' Administration Hospital, Mr. Alverti asked me, "Is life so sweet?" when I timidly used the white cane technique he was teaching me. I learned he really meant, "Let's step out, Miss Lovit. Let's show the world we can. Let's do things with strength and courage not worth doing otherwise." He lived that way. His example helped me to understand what I did and mastered would recharge me.

Mr. Ryan's charisma and dedication to doing a job right and to treating everyone with dignity and respect reemphasized this message. For me, his special magic was in building up my self-reliance! Although almost 45 years older than I, he seemed as much a contemporary as an elder. He could change his mind when he knew it was right to do so, but his values were constant. I grew from his example and encouragement and felt that I was accomplishing important work.

Frequently, there were humbling events and risky decisions to make that had uncertain consequences and challenges I wanted to avoid. But joy came over me when I experienced enthusiasm, energy, and willingness to do my best. Work in occupational therapy can be like an exotic banquet, offering tantalizing dishes to explore that in turn can lead into opportunities to create "recipes" or applications of one's own. Such an opportunity appeared for me and led me into the development of the Five-Stage Group Model.

Historically, therapeutic group work focused on spoken communication to express feelings about relationships and insights about clients' actions. However, group interventions for populations with some disabilities were never sufficiently explored. Some therapists assumed that people could not be included in a group session if they could not talk, did not understand language, could not understand how to play a game, or were confused or noisy. However, it is those populations that particularly need the socialization of a group; it is from the group that they receive necessary education and skills. I observed that each person in a group watched other members and, because each had different capabilities and strengths, they had something to show one another. I experimented with ways in which people could benefit from being connected in a group where speech was not the focus. Occupational therapy, with its emphasis on *doing*, brought me personal satisfaction and offered a way of meeting the challenges that go with testing the conventional wisdom.

Dr. Mihaly Csikszentmihalyi (1993, 2003) has written several books on the concept of *flow*. In *The Evolving Self*, he describes it as a "rare state of consciousness" (2003, xiii). He explains that flow is the experience of total concentration on a challenging task or an idea that cannot be achieved while one is being entertained or distracted. One must become actively and intensely involved in a difficult task to stretch the capacities. I wholeheartedly accepted the challenge of working with people with whom it was difficult to make a verbal connection.

Flow happened when I began to feel excited about getting clients to respond. I became convinced that the healing value of a group experience was necessary, and that it was my obligation to find the right method. One by one, the five stages evolved as one difficulty was met and another presented itself.

Relating to others nonverbally is very interesting. A connection made between two people without words is a golden moment, perhaps the more poignant because it appears so stark, so pure. These golden moments occurred whenever a group member showed new awareness. It happened, for example, when someone could share an unspoken idea with a group using an action. When I asked others to report on an act of kindness shown to them, one young woman, lacking speech, spread her fingers out to show her painted nails. It became clear she had a loving mother who had done this, as another member with very special verbal and inimitable gestures extracted this information. Another member learned for the first time to pass an item to another member. I saw it when one client with Alzheimer's disease suddenly intercepted a large soft ball before his male neighbor could reach it and then handed it to a withdrawn woman sitting next to him so she could have a turn. I remember seeing the golden moment in Jon, a young adult with Down syndrome whose psychological grade was age 1 year and who lacked all speech. During one group session, a bucket was pushed around from one member to another so that each could withdraw one item. As Jon reached for his item he noticed, remarkably, that the woman in the wheelchair next to him was trying unsuccessfully to pull her object from the bucket. Slowly, Jon reached down and pushed the bucket closer to her so that she could succeed. What one-year-old can produce such thoughtfulness?

The golden moment was observed in the sudden smile, the unconsciously straightened posture, or the unsolicited hug that came for the first time from someone who had previously avoided contact or response. When a string of such moments happened, a marvelous feeling occurred that illuminated my understanding of how to proceed. It was easy to become addicted to encouraging the feeling of flow.

Life is a constant surprise—work, personal life, and feelings are constantly in flux. To confront the upsetting surprises it is essential to form steadfast beliefs and values. And starting with meaningful work is a good way to begin. This can even help one weather settings where no peace exists. Organic life is expressed in an ebb and flow that is ever changing on its way to maturing or deteriorating and disappearing. This is so in personal events, in a bureaucracy, or in a profession. Knowing this, the "ebb" time can bring some understanding, patience, preparedness, and hope.

Even true tales have a fairy godmother or godfather, ogres, and magical times. And in every true story, there is the time to ride into the sunset.

I was walking along Sepulco Avenue in Los Angeles one Monday morning in June 1999 when I was overtaken with a feeling of tranquility. It had been a year since I had stopped having a planned schedule. Others call that time "retirement"; I called it "turning a corner." Although I was going in another direction, I was still reading occupational therapy literature, still engaged with my involved friends, and always ready to give a presentation or contribute to a book while planning how to integrate the past with the present and future. I acknowledged my satisfaction with and my keen delight in my three grown children who were responsible adults on their own. I now walked on an avenue free of past responsibilities.

I walked by a church that was bordered by gorgeous, large, multicolored roses. As I walked around the churchyard, I leaned closer to smell the flowers. There were spectacular varieties there, some in bud, some half-opened. I could hardly believe it, but all those beautiful roses lacked a scent.

Suddenly, at the back of the church, I noticed some large yellow roses that were fully opened and overgrown, as high as my shoulder. Some of the petals had brown and split edges. The mammoth bush was way past its prime; loose, rangy, and sagging. Yet the aroma of those older flowers was so strong, so full of an unabashedly pungent perfume, that it was in vibrant contrast to the others I had passed. I felt the joy of a sweet reward for persisting to explore the whole area.

The rewards of aging are the same. The flower acquiring the deepening *scent* by surviving is the same as the older person surviving and feeling satisfaction with life's experiences. It is my metaphor for gaining a keener, bolder *sense* of gratitude and of recognition for how I came to live in the space around me. It is filled with a liberating freedom of learning to expect the ebb and flow of events in life.

I want to remember that it is up to me to encourage the flow, and it is up to me to not lose heart too much when the ebb is there. Tapping into occupational therapy, I can know what to do. Reflecting on the people that came into my life can remind me how to be.

REFERENCES

American Board of Psychiatry and Neurology. (n.d.). *Mission and history.* Retrieved September 24, 2007, from http://www.abpn.com/mission.htm

American Occupational Therapy Association. (1985a, April). *Occupational therapy manpower: A plan for progress.* Rockville, MD: Author.

American Occupational Therapy Association. (1985b, July). Wilma West honored. *Occupational Therapy News, 39,* 1.

American Occupational Therapy Association. (1991). *Education data survey final report: Survey of 1990 educational programs.* Rockville, MD: Author.

American Occupational Therapy Association. (2004). *Definition of occupational therapy practice for the AOTA Model Practice Act.* Bethesda, MD: Author. (Available from the State Affairs Group, 4720 Montgomery Lane, Bethesda, MD 20814)

American Occupational Therapy Association. (2007). *Centennial Vision* and Executive Summary. *American Journal of Occupational Therapy, 61,* 613–614.

American Occupational Therapy Association. (2008). Occupational therapy practice framework: Domain and process (2nd ed.). *American Journal of Occupational Therapy, 62,* 625–683.

Americans with Disabilities Act, 42 U.S.C. § 12101 *et seq* (1990).

Armstrong, C. E. (1996). *The education of students with mental retardation in the United States.* Portales, NM: Eastern New Mexico University. (ERIC Document Reproduction Service No. ED395447)

Ayres, A. J. (1972). *Sensory integration and learning disorders.* Los Angeles: Western Psychological Services.

Ayres, A. J. (1979). *Sensory integration and the child.* Los Angeles: Western Psychological Services.

Ayres, A. J., Erwin, P. R., & Mailloux, Z. (2004). *Love, Jean: Inspiration for families living with dysfunction of sensory integration*. Santa Rosa, CA: Crestport.

Ayres, A. J., Henderson, A., Llorens, L., Gilfoyle, E., Myers, C., & Prevel, S. (1974). *The development of sensory integrative theory and practice: A collection of works of A. Jean Ayres*. Dubuque, IA: Kendall/Hunt.

Bailey, D. M. (1998). Legislative and reimbursement influences on occupational therapy: Changing opportunities. In M. E. Neistadt & E. B. Crepeau (Eds.), *Williard and Spackman's occupational therapy* (9th ed., pp. 763–771). Philadelphia: Lippincott.

Baker, P. (2007, May 28). Driver rehabilitation: Assessing the older driver. *OT Practice, 12*, 10–16.

Brachtesende, A. (2007, July 9). Member Forum—The *Centennial Vision* moving ahead to 2017. *OT Practice, 12*, 23–25.

Clark, F. (1993). Occupation embedded in a real life: Interweaving occupational science and occupational therapy. *American Journal of Occupational Therapy, 47*, 1067–1078.

Clark, F., Azen, S. P., Zemke, R., Jackson, J., Carlson, M., Mandel, D., et al. (1997). Occupational therapy for independent-living older adults. A randomized controlled trial. *Journal of the American Medical Association, 278*, 1321–1326.

Cole, M. B. (1998). *Group dynamics in occupational therapy: The theoretical basis and practice application of group treatment* (2nd ed.). Thorofare, NJ: SLACK.

Colmar, M. (1998, June 22). Making sense of prospective payment, terms, and definitions under the BBA. *Advance for Occupational Therapy Practitioners*, p. 27.

Cox, R. C., & West, W. L. (1982). *Fundamentals of research for health professionals*. Laurel, MD: Ramsco.

Csikszentmihalyi, M. (1993). *The evolving self: Psychology for the third millennium*. New York: Harper-Collins.

Csikszentmihalyi, M. (2003). *Good business, leadership, flow, and the making of meaning*. New York: Viking.

Diffendal, J. (1998, August 31). The OT job market: Does anyone know where it's going? *Advance for Occupational Therapy Practitioners*, p. 7.

Education of the Handicapped Act Amendments of 1986, P.L. 99–457, 100 Stat. 1145.

Education for all Handicapped Children Act, P.L. 94–142, 89 Stat 773 (1975).

Evanofski, M. (2003). Occupational therapy reimbursement, regulation, and the evolving scope of practice. In E. B. Crepeau, E. S. Cohen, & B. A. Boyt Schell (Eds.), *Willard and Spackman's occupational therapy* (10th ed., pp. 887–896). Baltimore: Lippincott Williams & Wilkins.

Family and Medical Leave Act, 29 U.S.C. § 28 (1993).

Fidler, G., & Fidler, J. (1964). *Occupational therapy: A communication process in psychiatry.* New York: Macmillan.

Fiorentino, M. (1963). *Reflex testing methods for evaluating CNS development.* Springfield, IL: Charles C Thomas.

Fiorentino, M. (1974). Occupational therapy: Realization to activation [Eleanor Clarke Slagle Lecture]. *American Journal of Occupational Therapy, 29,* 15–29.

Fiorentino, M. (1981). *A basis of sensorimotor development—Normal and abnormal: The influence of primitive, postural reflexes on the development and distribution of tone.* Springfield, IL: Charles C Thomas.

Foto, M. (1997). Nationally Speaking: Presidential Address—Wilma West: A true visionary. *American Journal of Occupational Therapy, 51,* 638–639.

Gillette, N. P. (1998). Dedication—A vision for the future. *American Journal of Occupational Therapy, 52,* 318–319.

Hasselkus, B. R. (2002). *The meaning of everyday occupation.* Thorofare, NJ: Slack.

Individuals with Disabilities Education Act Amendments, 34 C.F.R. Part 303 (1997).

Jackson, J., Carlson, M., Mandel, D., Zemke, R., & Clark, F. (1998). Occupation in lifestyle redesign: The well elderly study occupational therapy program. *American Journal of Occupational Therapy, 52,* 326–336.

Kavale, K. A. (2002). Mainstreaming to full inclusion: From orthogenesis to pathogenesis of an idea. *International Journal of Disability, Development, and Education, 49,* 201–214.

Kennedy, J. F. (1961, January 20). *Inaugural address.* Retrieved September 25, 2007, from www.presidency.ucsb.edu/ws/index.php?pid=8032

King, L. J. (1974). A sensory-integrative approach to schizophrenia. *American Journal of Occupational Therapy, 28,* 529–536.

Krauthamer, J. (2005, Fall/Winter). Class speaker: Janet Krauthamer, Class of 2005. *The Motivator: The Occupational Therapy Alumni Newsletter,* p. 6. Commencement address, Occupational Therapy Department, Columbia University, New York.

Kronenberg, F., Algado, S. S., & Pollard, N. (2005). *Occupational therapy without borders: Learning from the spirit of survivors.* Edinburgh, UK: Elsevier/Churchill Livingstone.

Law, M. (Ed.). (1998). *Client-centered occupational therapy.* Thorofare, NJ: Slack.

Lee, H. (1960). *To kill a mockingbird.* Philadelphia: J. B. Lippincott.

Llorens, L. A. (1969). Facilitating growth and development: The promise of occupational therapy [Eleanor Clarke Slagle Lecture]. *American Journal of Occupational Therapy, 24,* 93–101.

Llorens, L. A. (1976). *Application of developmental theory for health and rehabilitation.* Rockville, MD: American Occupational Therapy Association.

Lowen, A. (1966). *The betrayal of the body.* New York: MacMillan.

Mace, N. L., & Rabins, P.V. (1981). *The 36-hour day: A family guide to caring for persons with Alzheimer disease, related dementing illnesses, and memory loss in later life.* Baltimore: Johns Hopkins University Press.

Mosey, A. C. (1973). *Activities therapy.* New York: Raven Press.

Nelson, D. L. (1996). Why the profession of occupational therapy will flourish in the 21st century [Eleanor Clarke Slagle Lecture]. *American Journal of Occupational Therapy, 51,* 11–24.

Neistadt, M. E., & Crepeau, E. B. (1998). Environments for practice. In M. E. Neistadt & E. B. Crepeau (Eds.), *Willard and Spackman's occupational therapy* (9th ed., pp. 760–771). Philadelphia: Lippincott.

Nicholson, C. K. (1968). *Anthropology and education.* Columbus, OH: Merrill.

Nicholson, C. K. (1975). Learning and mental health. *Humanitas: Journal of the Institute of Man, 11,* 345–362.

Nicholson, C. K. & Nicholson, J. (Eds.). (1982). *The Personalized Care Model for the elderly* (2nd ed.). New York: Department of Hygiene.

Padilla, R. (2005a). Historical context [The 1950s]. In R. Padilla (Ed.), *A professional legacy: The Eleanor Clarke Slagle Lectures in Occupational Therapy, 1955–2004* (2nd ed., pp. 3–6). Bethesda, MD: AOTA Press.

Padilla, R. (2005b). Historical context [The 1960s]. In R. Padilla (Ed.), *A professional legacy: The Eleanor Clarke Slagle Lectures in Occupational Therapy, 1955–2004* (2nd ed., pp. 60–66). Bethesda, MD: AOTA Press.

Padilla, R. (2005c). Historical context [The 1970s]. In R. Padilla (Ed.), *A professional legacy: The Eleanor Clarke Slagle Lectures in Occupational Therapy, 1955–2004* (2nd ed., pp. 171–176). Bethesda, MD: AOTA Press.

Padilla, R. (2005d). Historical context [The 1990s]. In R. Padilla (Ed.), *A professional legacy: The Eleanor Clarke Slagle Lectures in Occupational Therapy, 1955–2004* (2nd ed., pp. 451–456). Bethesda, MD: AOTA Press.

Pakula, A. J. (Producer), & Mulligan, R. (Director). (1962). *To kill a mockingbird* [Motion Picture]. Los Angeles: Universal.

Peloquin, S. M. (2005). Embracing our ethos, reclaiming our heart [Eleanor Clarke Slagle Lecture]. *American Journal of Occupational Therapy, 59,* 611–625.

Ross, M. (1987). *Group process: Using therapeutic activities in chronic care.* Thorofare, NJ: Slack.

Ross, M. (1991). *Integrative group therapy: The structured five-stage approach* (2nd ed.). Thorofare, NJ: Slack.

Ross, M. (1997). *Integrative group therapy: Mobilizing coping abilities with the Five-Stage Group.* Bethesda, MD: AOTA Press.

Ross, M., & Bachner, S. (Eds.). (1998). *Adults with developmental disabilities: Current approaches in occupation therapy.* Bethesda, MD: AOTA Press.

Ross, M., & Bachner, S. (Eds.). (2004). *Adults with developmental disabilities: Current approaches in occupational therapy* (rev. ed.). Bethesda, MD: AOTA Press.

Ross, M., & Burdick, D. (1978). *A sensory integration training manual for regressed and geriatric psychiatric patients.* Middletown: Department of Rehabilitation Services, Connecticut Valley Hospital.

Ross, M., & Burdick, D. (1981). *Sensory integration: A training manual for therapists and teachers for regressed, psychiatric and geriatric patient groups.* Thorofare, NJ: Slack.

Siebert, C. (2003, May 5). Aging in place: Implications for occupational therapy, *OT Practice, 8,* CE1–CE8.

Smith, E. W. L. (Ed.). (1976) *The growing edge of Gestalt therapy.* New York: Brunner/Mazel.

Social Security Act, P.L. 89–97 (1965).

Steib, P. A. (1998, September 10). Views from the top: Major rehab players jockey for position. *OT Week, 12,* 12–13, 15–16.

Struthers, M. S., & Boyt Schell, B. (1991). Public policy and its influence on performance. In C. Christiansen & C. Baum (Eds.), *Occupational therapy: Overcoming human performance deficits* (pp. 178–196). Thorofare, NJ: Slack.

Tomes, N. (1994). *The art of asylum-keeping: Thomas Story Kirkbride and the origins of American psychiatry.* Philadelphia: University of Pennsylvania Press.

Torrey, E. F. (1997). *Out of the shadows: Confronting America's mental illness crisis.* New York: John Wiley & Sons.

West. W. L. (1958). The present status of graduate education in occupational therapy. *American Journal of Occupational Therapy, 12,* 291–292, 299.

West, W. L. (1976). Nationally Speaking—Research seminar. *American Journal of Occupational Therapy, 30,* 477–478.

West, W. L. (1982). The Foundation—Message from the President: The need, the response: *Occupational Therapy Journal of Research. American Journal of Occupational Therapy, 35,* 44.

West, W. L. (1989). Nationally Speaking—Perspectives on the past and future, part 1. *American Journal of Occupational Therapy, 43,* 787–790.

West, W. L. (1990). Nationally Speaking—Perspectives on the past and future, part 2. *American Journal of Occupational Therapy, 44,* 9–10.

West, W. L. (1992). Ten milestone issues in AOTA history. *American Journal of Occupational Therapy, 46,* 1066–1074.

U.S. Department of Justice. (2005). *A guide to disability rights laws.* Washington, DC: Author. Retrieved September 18, 2007, from www.usdoj.gov/crt/ada/cguide.htm

Untermeyer, L. (Ed.). (1971). *Robert Frost's poems.* New York: Washington Square Press.

Yalom, I. D. (1983). *Inpatient group psychotherapy.* New York: Basic Books.

APPENDIX

After graduating from a private university's occupational therapy program, in Hamden, Connecticut, in 1975, I never imagined the scope of my practice over the past 33 years would extend to 6 of the 7 continents. My clinical practice focused on adults with neurological disorders before I made a transition to teaching in 1988. The rigors of teaching occupational therapy students in the United States offers one type of experience; teaching in a developing country offers a completely different experience. My early assignments took me to China in 1995 and 1997 thanks to the support of the World Health Organization on both occasions. In 1997, eight occupational therapy students participated in a fieldwork opportunity that was my first of many attempts to encourage students to consider new emerging global practice areas. Since that time, I have developed many more opportunities in countries such as Costa Rica, Barbados, Bangladesh, South Africa, and Guatemala. Promoting global partnerships and multicultural communication resulted in my award to the AOTA Roster of Fellows in June 2003.

One does not need to travel to developing nations in order to learn about "diversity." International short courses were designed and offered students travel to the United Kingdom and Australia. My support for the World Federation of Occupational Therapy (WFOT) included encouraging students to attend the Congress that occurs every four years; as such, Quinnipiac University students and faculty attended and participated in the Congress in United Kingdom (1994), Montreal (1998), Sweden (2002), and Australia (2006). I look forward to WFOT Congress in Chile (2010) and Japan (2014).

My belief in international growth experiences and my attempts to foster such exchanges for students has led me to partner with the Schweitzer Institute. David Ives, Director of the Schweitzer Institute, has collaborated with me to sponsor occupational therapy students via financial support of their visits to countries in Central America. Furthermore he has engaged and supported my academic colleagues in Central America to travel to the United States as presenters at Quinnipiac University for international conferences with health-related themes.

My university supports international outreach, as evidenced by my receipt of Galpin International Fellowship Award. I was the first faculty member to receive this award in 2005. This allowed me to travel and teach in Bangladesh at the Health Professions Institute of the Center for the Rehabilitation of the Paralyzed. I serve on the International Education Advisory Board at Quinnipiac University and was awarded in 2003 the International Scholar, Phi Beta Delta Epsilon Theta Chapter. I received in 2002 an international grant that provided funding to explore the development of a short course in Costa Rica.

In 2008, as an AOTA elected second alternate delegate to WFOT, I traveled to Ljubljana, Slovenia. Some of the delegates who also attended the WFOT council meeting were prominent therapists I had met while teaching and supervising students in other countries. Seeing familiar faces in Slovenia—who could have imagined that 33 years ago. The occupational therapy students of Ljubljana helped host the council meeting. Like students everywhere around the world today, they are anxious to learn about other peoples in new environments. Eagerness to seek out diversity seems to be a universal goal of young students. Occupational therapy students whom I encounter demonstrate a strong desire to travel and discover new lands. I believe that we need to envision a future with the development of occupational therapy on a global scale to meet the needs of the citizens of the world.

— **Signian McGeary, MS, OTR/L, FAOTA**
   Assistant Professor, Quinnipiac University
   Past President, Connecticut Occupational Therapy Association
   USA 2nd Alternate Delegate, World Federation of Occupational Therapists

INDEX

A

Adults with Developmental Disabilities: Current Approaches in Occupational Therapy (Ross and Bachner), 84

Alverti, Peter, 12–13, 103

American Occupational Therapy Association (AOTA)
        award to Ross, 113
        vision of West, 32–33

American Occupational Therapy Foundation (ATOF), 32

arts, importance in behavioral health, 29–30

Ascher, Karoline, 42

Ashkins, Ellen, 54

awards and honors, 65–66, 113–114

Ayres, A. Jean, 33, 38, 40–41

B

behavioral health, 27–30, 91–96

Binderman, Mary, 33

blind, work with, 11–27

Boccacio, Dolores, 58–59

Bronx Veteran's Hospital, 11–13

Brown, Marcus, 79

Burdick, Dona, 54–55

C

cane travel, 12–13, 15

Carlson, Lois, 35

Caudle, Adele, 28

Cedarcrest Hospital, 39–45

client groups. *see* group sessions

clients
        learning from, 73–75
        role of, 39–40

Cole, Marilyn, 83

Undercliff Hospital position, 28–30
work with the blind, 11–27
workshops by, 71
Ryan, Stetson K., 13–15, 26–27, 103–104

S
school setting, working in, 69–70
Schweitzer Institute, 114
Scott, Anne, 71
sensory integration, 38, 40–41
sheltered workshops, 37
Simpson, Dorothea, 17–18
Smaga, Brenda, 51–54
Small, Janet, 35
state institutions, nature of, 68
state psychiatric hospital position, 98–101
Steward, Barbara (Bobby), 34

T
To Kill a Mockingbird (Lee), 66–67

U
Undercliff Hospital, 28–30

V
veterans, special needs of, 11–12

W
West, Wilma L., vision of, 32–33
work services, 71–72
workshops, 37, 71

ABOUT THE AUTHOR

Mildred Ross, OTR/L, FAOTA, has practiced as an occupational therapist since her graduation from Columbia University in 1951. She has conducted more than 100 presentations on the Five-Stage Group Model, a strategy she has developed and discussed in six books and many articles. She most recently co-edited *Adults With Developmental Disabilities: Current Approaches in Occupational Therapy, Revised Edition,* with Susan Bachner (2004, AOTA Press).